Chakra Yoga

CHAKRA YOGA

*Balancing Energy
for Physical, Spiritual,
and Mental Well-Being*

ALAN FINGER

WITH KATRINA REPKA

SHAMBHALA
Boston & London
2005

SHAMBHALA PUBLICATIONS, INC.
Horticultural Hall
300 Massachusetts Avenue
Boston, Massachusetts 02115
www.shambhala.com

9 8 7 6 5 4

Printed in the United States of America

♾ This edition is printed on acid-free paper that meets
the American National Standards Institute z39.48 Standard.
♻ Shambhala Publications makes every effort to print on recycled paper.
For more information please visit www.shambhala.com.
Distributed in the United States by Random House, Inc.,
and in Canada by Random House of Canada Ltd

Library of Congress Cataloging-in-Publication Data
Finger, Alan, 1946–
Chakra yoga: balancing energy for physical, spiritual, and
mental well-being / Alan Finger and Katrina Repka.—1st ed.
p. cm.
Includes bibliographical references.
ISBN 978-1-59030-255-2 (pbk.: alk. paper)
1. Hatha yoga. 2. Chakras. I. Repka, Katrina. II. Title.
RA781.7.F558 2005
613.7'046—dc22
2005007962

CONTENTS

Preface   *vii*

Acknowledgments   *xiii*

INTRODUCTION: WHAT IS YOGA?   1

1. WHAT ARE THE CHAKRAS?   7

2. FINDING ROOTS ∼ *Muladhara, the Earth Chakra*   19

3. DISCOVERING FLOW ∼ *Svadhishthana, the Water Chakra*   37

4. ILLUMINATING GEMS ∼ *Manipura, the Fire Chakra*   53

5. HARMONIZING EMOTIONS ∼ *Anahata, the Air Chakra*   71

6. COMMUNICATING WITH YOUR SPIRIT ∼ *Vishuddha, the Space Chakra*   85

7. ACCESSING YOUR INTUITION ∼ *Ajna Chakra, Commander of the Elements*   99

8. Radiating Power ⁓ *Sahasrara Chakra, beyond the Elements*   115

9. Mantra and Yantra   121

10. A Final Word of Encouragement   127

    Appendix: Putting It All Together   129

    Resources   139

PREFACE

I HAVE BEEN LIVING and teaching yoga for more than forty years, and it is a great pleasure to share some of my knowledge in this book on the chakra system. The chakras are the body's seven main physical, mental, and spiritual centers; together they form the pathway to healing, rejuvenation, and growth.

The chakras govern many things: relationships, creativity, personal power and magnetism, emotions, communication, intuition, and the ability to access divine wisdom. It does not matter how old you are or whether you have prior yoga experience, you can use the chakras to attain balance—a state of harmony and equilibrium—in all areas of your life. Through the chakra system I have transformed my own life and seen compelling changes in the lives of many others. To me, the chakras are an indispensable framework for self-exploration.

MY HISTORY WITH YOGA

I was born in 1946 in Johannesburg, South Africa. Mani, my father, had fought in the Second World War and suffered from shell shock. He turned to drugs and alcohol to cope with the severe anxiety and nervous disorder associated with his trauma. His struggles with addiction, and the burdens they placed on our family, are what I remember of my early childhood.

After many attempts to find my father a cure, my grandfather, who was a prominent businessman in South Africa, encouraged him to get more involved in the family business. He thought that if my father became absorbed in something other than his "madnesses," as my grandfather called them, the addictions would fall away. One of my grandfather's businesses, Liberty Imports, involved the trade of goods between South Africa and the United States. He sent my father on a buying trip to Los Angeles that changed his life.

In Los Angeles, my father stayed at the famous Ambassador Hotel, where Paramahansa Yogananda, one of the most prominent yogis of the twentieth century and author of *Autobiography of a Yogi*, happened to be giving a lecture. My father had never heard of Yogananda, but something compelled him to go. The lecture had such a powerful effect on my father that he asked to meet with Yogananda later in private. In their meeting, Yogananda foretold that both my father and one of his two sons would devote their lives to teaching yoga. My brother Ron became a businessman, and I a yogi.

Following Yogananda's counsel, my father headed to India on the first of many trips devoted to the intensive study of yoga that would continue for the rest of his life. He went to the Sivananda ashram in Rishikesh and also visited Yogananda's brother, Bishnu Gosh. My father returned to South Africa when I was five. He had conquered his addictions and from then on became a full-time yogi and teacher. Our household became a virtual ashram; each year we hosted many of the leading Indian swamis and yogis who came to South Africa to teach.

However, the difficult early years with my father had left their mark on me. At fifteen I weighed 265 pounds and was a compulsive eater. I was doing poorly in school and suffered from terrible anxiety and heart palpitations. My parents decided to send me to a psychiatrist. During the session, I noticed that this therapist couldn't contain his nervous energy and anxiety: he was continually twitching, tapping his foot, and shifting in his seat—and he was a chain smoker! This experience made me even more depressed, for it seemed the therapist was more neurotic than I was. I did not return. Instead, knowing how yoga had helped my father, I decided to give it a try.

My father was reluctant to teach me at first, because we were family. Rather than instruct me, he preferred that I join him in his yoga and meditation practice as an equal. Like the ancient rishis, he believed that the universe would guide me; I would absorb everything by watching and copying, and the wisdom would be transferred naturally.

Once I decided to practice with my father, he would wake me in the morning by flicking my bedroom light on and off twice—at 4:30 A.M. At first it was hard to get up; there were many days when I would have preferred to continue dozing. But over time, I discovered for myself the benefits of yoga: I lost one hundred pounds in just three months and eliminated my self-destructive and compulsive tendencies. My anxiety went away and I became strong and clear in thought and action. The world began to reveal its wonders to me.

Over the years, my father and I together studied with a number of different teachers. We became very close with Swami Venkatesananda, who spent three months of each year living at our house. Venkatesananda came from the Sivananda ashram in India and was known as Sivananda's "jewel student." Like Yogananda, Sivananda was a great yogi. He taught authentic classical yoga to thousands of followers and sent his top students to disseminate his teachings in the West: Swami Satchitananda founded Integral Yoga in the United States, Swami Vishnudevananda founded the International Sivananda Yoga Vedanta Centers in Canada and Australia, and Swami Venkatesananda came to us in South Africa.

Venkatesananda was the translator of many Sanskrit works on yoga and brought with him a huge wealth of knowledge: asana, *kriya* (the yoga of purifying consciousness) and *laya* (the yoga of meditative absorption), yoga philosophy, ayurveda (the Indian science of life), and the *Yoga Sutras*. He was one of my most powerful influences. When I was twenty, Venkatesananda initiated me into the higher teachings and gave me the title Yogiraj (Master of Yoga) and the name Yogi Amrita. He also taught me *shakti pat*, which is a transmission of energy

handed down from teacher to student that gives the student the experience of other states of consciousness.

My father and I also studied with Swami Nisreyasananda, who was from the Rama Krishna lineage. He introduced us to Tantra, a spiritual philosophy devoted to the quest for liberation, and was the first teacher to emphasize that the way one lives one's life is the ultimate gauge of spirituality. In Tantra, you do not need to adopt a dogma or tattoo OM symbols on your body in order to be a yogi. Rather, you must strive to use everyday experience as a means to spiritual realization. Nisreyasananda was originally an engineer and had a very structured, scientific approach to yoga; he taught us everything from yoga philosophy to mantra. Nisreyasananda also showed us how the *nadi*s (energy meridians in the body) relate to the physical practice of asanas and explained how certain elements of yoga are based on scientific ratios and formulas. (In Sanskrit, the plural of *asana* is the same as the singular. In an English-language context, we are making it plural by adding *s* to conform to current usage.) One time he broke down the iconography of the elephant god Ganesha into a circle, a triangle, and a square, which he then related to structural principles of engineering. Although some of what he taught was hard for me to grasp, he was fascinating.

Our learning was advanced with Master Bharati, who initiated my father and me more fully into Tantra. Bharati was a poet who had gone into a cave for many years of contemplation and then decided that seclusion was not the way to yoga. Realizing that we all must evolve together, he came down from the mountains to immerse himself in the study of Tantra. Before Bharati, I was consumed with the idea that in order to fully live and teach yoga I had to become a monk and practice *brahmacharya* (sexual abstinence as laid out in the Hindu writings). He reassured me that the yoga my father and I were practicing, and how we were living, was the essence of Tantra and that it didn't require a monastic way of life. Bharati taught Tantra as a science that could lead toward liberation on this plane of consciousness.

When B. K. S. Iyengar was young and not yet well known, he too came to South Africa to give workshops and lectures. We studied with him when his book *Light on Yoga* was first published, and we became familiar with his approach to the physical practice of asanas. Iyengar had perfected the concept of form and alignment, which brought a new dimension to the way my father and I trained our bodies.

Each of these teachers had much to offer. Over many years, my father and I assimilated their knowledge and integrated it into our own practice and teachings. This led us to develop our own system, ISHTA yoga, which is founded on the belief that the best yoga is one that is tailored to individual needs and circumstances.

ISHTA YOGA

ISHTA is an acronym that stands for the Integrated Sciences of Hatha (practices designed to balance the polarities in each individual), Tantra and Ayurveda. ISHTA also evokes the Sanskrit word *ishta*, which means "individual" or "personalized." Underlying ISHTA yoga is the belief that every person who practices yoga needs an individualized daily practice to keep happy and healthy. This practice is called *ishta sadhana*, or "individual means of realization." In the *Yoga Sutras*, verse 2.44 states: "*svadhyaya istadevate samprayogah.*" This means that through self-study one discovers one's individual path to spiritual enlightenment. In the Hindu tradition, an individual deity, or *ishta devata*, is given by a teacher to a student in order to foster personal growth. The deity is chosen because it symbolizes certain qualities that the student needs to work on. We developed ISHTA in order to give every individual a unique practice based on his or her physical constitution and way of life.

COMING TO AMERICA

After teaching in South Africa for thirteen years, I decided to emigrate to the United States in 1975. My brother had already made that move and encouraged me to join him. After traveling around for a few months, I settled in Los Angeles with my wife and two children. At first I thought I would look for work as a photographer and visited various photography studios. One day I was talking to a potential client when a few of his friends arrived. It came up that I taught yoga, and they asked me to teach them. I did, and they loved it! Word spread, and within a few months I was driving all over LA teaching yoga. I ended up with celebrities such as Robin Williams, Barbra Streisand, Neil Diamond, Joni Mitchell, and Diana Ross as my students. In 1988 I founded Yoga Works in Santa Monica, California. My goal was to create a modern studio environment where yoga could be taught in an upbeat, vital way.

In 1993 I sold my interest in Yoga Works, moved to New York City, where I live today, and founded Yoga Zone (which later became Be Yoga), with four studios in and around Manhattan. In 2004 Be Yoga was bought by Yoga Works, which has me reunited with my original partners in Los Angeles!

What This Book Is About

The purpose of this book is to illustrate, as clearly as possible, some of the deeper concepts of ISHTA yoga, as they relate to the physical, mental, and spiritual practice. Specifically focused on the chakras, the following chapters will provide you with knowledge and practical exercises to use to create positive change in your life, suited to your individual needs and circumstances.

I have seen how yoga works to effect deep personal growth. It transformed my father, me, and many of our students. It has also connected us to divine intuition, inspiration, and insight—what I call the "in" things. One of the great joys of my life has been sharing yoga with others. To me the success of your yoga practice is not measured by how well you can do the poses or how long you can sit and meditate. It is measured by how well you are living your life. Ask yourself: Do I feel there is a balance in my life and harmony in my relations with others? Can I experience unconditional love? Am I fulfilling my needs from the abundance of the universe? Am I happy just to be alive?

Use this book as a tool to help you answer yes to these important questions. Although working on yourself can be a great challenge, there are many rewards to be had, even if you can only manage to do a little each day. Start slowly, and gradually the unconditional love, abundance, and happiness that you discover within will spill over into every moment of your life!

HARI OM, OM TAT SAT

"Immerse yourself in unconditional love and saturate yourself in unlimited consciousness."

I am grateful that you have chosen to read my book. Together, let us start a journey of transformation.

ACKNOWLEDGMENTS

THANKS TO my father and all of the teachers in the ISHTA lineage who initiated me and gave me the means to share this amazing information with others.

Thanks to all of the wonderful teachers in the ISHTA community who are continuing the tradition in North America, as well as Rachel Zinman-Jeanes and Kumiko Mack, who have introduced the ISHTA teachings to Australia and Japan, respectively.

Thanks to Beverley Murphy, Kara Sekular, and Chris Grey for help with details of the manuscript, and Jenny Aurthur for her visual style with the photos. Thanks to our agent, Jodi Weiss, who championed this project from the beginning. And to Emily Bower and all of the staff at Shambhala.

Finally, special thanks to Katrina, for bringing this book to fruition.

Hari Om,
Alan

Thanks to my family, for all that they have given me; to Alan, for his wisdom and inspiration; and to Chris, always.

Namaste,
Katrina

CHAKRA YOGA

INTRODUCTION
What Is Yoga?

To action alone are you entitled, never to its fruit.
Let not the fruit of action be your motive.
Neither let there be any attachment to inaction.

Abiding in yoga, do your work without attachment
And with being balanced in success or failure.
Balance is called yoga.
    —*The Bhagavad Gita*

YOGA IS A TREE with many branches. It is a physical practice that consists of specific postures to realign and strengthen the body. It is a mental practice that incorporates breath work and meditation. And it is a spiritual practice: yoga integrates the body and mind and reconnects you to your own perfection. The word *yoga* comes from the Sanskrit root *yuj,* which means "to yoke" or "to harness." Yoga describes the experience of uniting the material self with the supreme intelligence of the universe, which brings unbounded joy, peace, and balance.

We all need balance. Balance brings healing. When you find balance, it mends body, mind, and spirit. A harmonious relationship must exist among the three in order to find happiness amid the pressures of daily life. Your balance may be affected by any of the following:

1

- muscular tension
- injury
- poor skeletal alignment
- toxic environments (physical, mental, spiritual)
- allergies
- noise pollution
- dealing with difficult people
- dissatisfaction with work, family, or finances
- negative thinking

All of these cause physical, mental, and spiritual disunity. The truth is that at your core you are already whole and in balance. You contain the knowledge of everything in the universe—all you need to do is find it within. It is like looking for your sunglasses: You search under the table, in the car, on the porch; you drive yourself to distraction trying to find them. Then suddenly you look in the mirror and see that they have been sitting on your head the whole time! They were never lost. In the same way, the higher intelligence that exists in the universe is always close at hand—if you know where to look. When you are able to connect to it, you find that the union that you have been searching for has always been there, waiting for you to discover it.

We are all drops of water from the great ocean of consciousness (Brahman). In every being exists a spirit (atman) that embodies the perfection of the universe. This perfection comprises infinite intelligence, happiness, clarity, and a profound sense of equilibrium. Imbalances occur when you become detached from your natural perfection; to find balance you must go within and reconnect with your spirit so that you can let its abundance spill over into your life.

THE PHYSICAL PRACTICE

Most people are familiar with yoga as a physical practice. A physical yoga practice consists of various postures, or asanas, that are linked together to strengthen, stretch, and realign the body. Each asana requires careful attention to body and breath. If done with conscious awareness, the asanas bring clarity to the mind and a sense of well-being to the body. The physical practice can bring numerous benefits:

- long, lean muscles
- improved posture and breathing
- realignment of the skeletal system
- enhanced digestion
- better circulation
- a relaxed nervous system
- greater immunity

The postures also give an internal massage to the organs, tissues, and muscles. They heal the body from the inside out.

It is in the body that you can begin to find balance, a principle in yoga called Hatha. *Ha* is the energy of the sun (*surya*); it is heat and power. *Tha* is the energy of the moon (*chandra*), which is coolness and flexibility. These two syllables together represent the balance between strength and relaxation that exists in every living thing, including plants (during the day they extend upward to absorb the sun's rays; at night they droop and soften).

In the physical practice of yoga, Ha represents the strengthening of your musculature, Tha the relaxation. There is a continuous play of Ha and Tha throughout your body and even in your nervous system, which reacts to passing phases of consciousness (conscious, subconscious, or unconscious), causing some parts of your body to contract and tighten and others to relax. For example, thinking too much causes stiffness in the neck and head; excessive emotion is felt in the heart and navel area (butterflies, or heaviness of heart). If there is stress in your unconscious, it is felt behind the legs, which is why people who don't do any exercise can still have tight legs. They get stiffness from tension in the unconscious mind.

Hatha yoga teaches you to strengthen areas of weakness and reduce tension in areas that are contracted. It is composed of a variety of asanas—standing poses, forward bends, backward bends, twists, and inversions—designed to create balance in every part of the body. This balance brings a feeling of lightness, space, strength, and union of opposites: yoga!

THE MENTAL PRACTICE

In addition to being a great physical practice, yoga is also a mental discipline. In each pose you must focus on your breath. You must also bring awareness to the way your muscles are working and the alignment of your body. The challenge is to keep your mind still and calm when your body feels fatigued or when you are distracted by outside thoughts. Practicing the postures requires an attention to detail that does not allow much room for you to think about what you are going to have for dinner, the fight you had with your spouse, or how much longer you have before practice is finished. If you are able to use the physical practice to draw your mind inward, the poses become a moving meditation. The physical practice also helps to work out tension in your body so that you can then sit comfortably in seated meditation and explore the deeper mental aspects of yoga.

Seated meditation has been shown to be helpful to people suffering from numerous diseases and imbalances in the body, including chronic pain, unexplained fatigue, addictions, headaches, high blood pressure, cardiovascular disease, anxiety disorders, and depression.

In order to understand how meditation works to bring balance and healing, it is important to recognize that there are two kinds of intelligence: a mind intelligence and a higher intelligence. Whereas in the West we tend to think of the mind as inhabiting the brain, in yoga these intelligences exist in every cell of the body. Your mind intelligence thinks, plans, and executes day-to-day activities; your higher intelligence uses the intelligence of the universe to keep your system in balance. Just as the seed of a fruit contains all the genetic information about the fruit itself, your higher intelligence contains the blueprint for your health and well-being. When your mind intelligence is overactive, it overrides the ability of your higher intelligence to keep you healthy and strong, and you fall prey to imbalance and disease. In order to stay healthy and balanced, you must calm your mental processes so that your higher intelligence may emerge.

Imagine your mind as a lake. When the water is disturbed and choppy, the bottom can't be seen. But when the water is calm and clear, you can see everything that lies beneath the surface. Similarly, if your mind is perturbed, your higher intelligence is obscured. Stilling the mind permits your higher intelligence to shine through.

Tantrikas (those who practice Tantra) use meditation to apply the balance of Hatha to the chakras. In the online audio meditations that accompany this book, I will teach you how to get in touch with the unique qualities and characteristics of each chakra and to balance your chakras in meditation. This will take you deeper to experience the profound healing and oneness that is at the core of your being and will in turn bring harmony into all areas of your life.

THE SPIRITUAL PRACTICE

Once you have balanced the chakras physically and mentally, it is possible to transcend material limitations and realize oneness with the divine energy of the universe, which in yoga is called *samadhi* (ecstasy or bliss). In Tantra, a belief in God or a supreme being is not necessary for studying yoga, nor does the study of yoga preclude specific religious beliefs. All people, regardless of religious affiliation, can benefit from having a healthier body and a clearer mind. If you wish to continue to tap into the subtle energy that exists in concert with your physical and mental selves, it will eventually lead you to a connection with the spiritual wisdom of the universe.

You may choose to begin your exploration of the chakras through the physical practice of yoga. Over time, you will probably find that your muscle tone will improve, your body will feel lighter, and your aches and pains will diminish. Perhaps you will stay with the physical practice for a number of months, or even years, before you get the urge to go deeper and meditate. Many of my most advanced students started off with no interest in the meditative aspects of yoga at all, but over the years they have benefited so much from the physical practice that they want to explore the meditative side. If you are just starting out on your journey, don't feel that you have to jump in all at once. Take your time and build your practice gradually. If you are already eager to learn meditation, remember that it takes time and discipline to train your mind. I advise you to try to practice a little bit every day. Even if your mind jumps around and brings up old emotions, thought patterns, and memories, just stick with it. Eventually, your mind will settle down long enough for you to get a glimpse of the bliss and spiritual connection that exists beyond it. Remember, the journey is not about the destination; it is about enjoying the trip.

I believe that the physical, mental, and spiritual aspects of the chakra system make it a fully comprehensive structure for self-study. In this book, I will show you how to use the chakras to explore all three aspects of your yoga practice and tailor them to your unique personality and circumstances. This journey will take you deep within yourself to experience the balance and union that is yoga.

ONE

WHAT ARE THE CHAKRAS?

WHAT EXACTLY are chakras? We see people wearing their symbols on sweaters and talking about them in yoga classes and over coffee, but we don't get the full picture of where they are, what they do, and how we can tune in to them so that we can make them real in our lives. In order to understand the chakras, it is important to understand how they are created and how each chakra comes to have its own individual qualities and characteristics. This chapter will explore the philosophical background of the chakras, give you a sense of where each chakra is located, and discuss how the different chakras function in your life.

The story of the chakras begins with the story of creation. Over the millennia there have been many different attempts to explain the phenomenon of existence, from the Bible to the big bang theory. My teachers explained the origins of the universe and the creation of humanity through two primary philosophies that have been handed down through the generations: Tantra and Samkhya.

Tantra explores the essential unity of reality. Samkhya analyzes the different elements of physical manifestation and explains how they take form from spirit. Tantra and Samkhya emerged around 350 to 500 C.E., although as with most Indian philosophies dating back as far as the Vedas of around 4000 B.C.E. to 2000 B.C.E., scholars debate over exact dates and timelines.*

* Georg Feuerstein, *The Yoga Tradition: Its History, Literature, Philosophy and Practice* (Prescott, Ariz.: Hohm Press, 2001), p. 96.

I have accumulated the wisdom of Tantra and Samkhya over many years from many different teachers, most of whom handed down this information orally. In the following discussion I have set down the essential components of Tantra and Samkhya as they were taught to me, in order to provide a framework that will help you better understand the chakras.

TANTRA

In Tantra, the creation of the universe is explained through the dynamic interplay of two powerful forces: Shiva and Shakti. Together, Shiva and Shakti represent ultimate reality and the union of all duality. By duality I mean that everything in the material universe is made up of opposites: light/dark, soft/loud, male/female, active/passive. Ultimate reality can be equated to the concept of a higher spirit that is beyond these opposites and the limited perception of our mind and senses. There are many things that we are unable to perceive. For example, radio waves and microwaves exist even though we cannot see them; many animals can hear and smell things that we can't. According to Tantra, the same applies to spirit: we may not be able to perceive it with our senses, but it is always there.

Shiva represents the male principle of nonfragmented consciousness and holds all of the knowledge of the universe. Shakti is the female principle of creative energy, equivalent to Mother Nature.

According to Tantra, Shiva/Shakti hold all dualities and opposites in a state of absolute unity on the plane of infinite consciousness, beyond our earthly concepts of time and space. To create our finite universe, Shiva and Shakti moved away from each other, releasing consciousness (*citta*) and energy (*prana*). Within consciousness there is *sat-cit-ananda: sat* is pure consciousness, *cit* is awareness of consciousness, and *ananda* is the experience of consciousness that requires a human form to become physically evident. Sat and cit continue to exist on the infinite plane; ananda manifests consciousness in the physical world.

After citta and prana are released to manifest conscious reality on the finite plane, maya (the illusory part of existence) occurs. Maya is the field of consciousness readily available to us in the world of the senses (sound, touch, sight, taste, smell), which we believe to be all that exists. Because of maya, we experience a total separation of Shiva and Shakti and conceive of the world in terms of duality, which is our way of making sense of existence. For example, to understand hot we need to experience cold; to appreciate light we need to be familiar with dark. Tantrikas believe that because maya does not let us experience the union of Shiva and Shakti, it causes us to lose connection with the divine and is therefore the source of human suffering.

The purpose of the tantric path is to realize through experience that the world of duality is only an illusion and that everything is divine and connected. Shiva and Shakti are never fully separate, and when we can realize that, we come to see the divine in all things.

SAMKHYA

Traditionally, the chakra system comes from tantric philosophy, which I will explore further, but first I would like to give a brief overview of Samkhya philosophy. Samkhya is one of the six *astika,* or Hindu philosophical schools of India, and is regarded as the oldest of Hinduism's orthodox philosophical systems. The sage Kapila is considered the founder of the Samkhya school, although no historical verification is possible. The definitive text of classical Samkhya is the *Samkhya-Karika,* written by Ishvara Krishna, circa 400–500 C.E. The word *Samkhya* literally means "number" and refers to the twenty-four (sometimes enumerated as twenty-five) processes that happen when a physical being is created. Samkhya helps to explain to us how matter is manifested from the intelligence of spirit.*

In Samkhya, *parusha* and *prakriti* are the terms that correlate to Tantra's Shiva and Shakti. According to Samkhya, when a spirit (atman) chooses a human birth in order to work out the karma attached to it, parusha and prakriti move apart to create a physical manifestation.** Prakriti (Mother Nature) contains all of the knowledge of the universe; it stores the blueprint for manifestation and karmic composition of each living thing as *mahat.* Once mahat is established, the next thing that is required is identity, which is called *ahamkara.* Ahamkara is the I-ness or feeling of self that you need in order to function in the world and identify yourself as separate from others. To hold identity in a body, there are three forces of movement, or *guna*s: *rajas, tamas,* and *sattva.* Rajas is the active force, tamas is the passive force, and sattva is a balance between the two. Everything in the universe contains a mixture of the three gunas: mind, intellect, ego, trees, plants, animals, and so on. In some forms of matter, the sattva guna predominates, in others rajas or tamas. For example, a stone,

---

* Dates for Samkhya are slightly problematic. According to Feuerstein (among others), 400–500 C.E. is the likely period when the *Samkhya-Karika,* the seminal text of classical Samkhya was composed. Kapila, who is also credited with authorship of the *Samkhya-Sutra,* is said by some scholars to have lived in the Vedic age; others place him much later (1300–1400 C.E.). See Feuerstein, *The Yoga Tradition,* p. 75.

** Karma is discussed in more detail in chapter 7.

being passive and inert, is full of tamas. The sun's rays, active and radiant, are more rajasic. The preponderance of a particular guna and the gunas in combination are what give things their particular attributes.

Once parusha and prakriti separate, and our blueprint of intelligence (mahat) and identity (ahamkara, which contains the three gunas) are established, we need a mind (*manas*) in order to manifest ourselves in the physical world. For manas to function, it needs a body and five senses. The body is made up of five elements (*bhuta*s): earth, water, fire, air, and space. Each element has a sense (*tanmatra*) associated with it, as well as an organ of knowledge (*jnana indriya*) through which it experiences the world, and an organ of action (*karma indriya*) that reacts to worldly experiences. The organs of knowledge are what the senses use to perceive the world; the organs of action are what the senses use to act on or as a result of what they perceive. Parusha, prakriti, mahat, ahamkara, manas, the five elements, the five senses, and the ten associated organs constitute the categories enumerated by Samkhya.

Because smells come from the constituents of earth, the sense for the earth element is smell. The organ of knowledge, or area of knowledge, for the earth element is the nose, which we use to smell the constituents of earth. The organ of action is the anus, which creates smell as it rids the body of excess earth in our system and regulates the amount of earth in us.

Water is associated with the sense of taste, because without water there is no taste; imagine trying to taste something without saliva in your mouth. The organ of knowledge is the tongue, which we use to taste. The organ, or area, of action is the genital region and bladder, which rid the body of excess water and regulate the amount of water in our system.

Fire gives light so that we can see, so its sense is sight. The organs of knowledge are the eyes, through which we see. The organs of action are the feet, because they react to what the eyes see.

The sense associated with air is touch. The organ of knowledge is the skin, through which we perceive air temperature and other stimuli, and experience sensation. The organ of action is the fingers, through which we touch others.

Space is associated with sound because sound carries over space. The ears are the organs of knowledge, as they process sound. The vocal cords are the organs of action, as they communicate sound over space.

This is how Samkhya philosophy explains the creation of matter from spirit.

THE CHAKRAS WITHIN TANTRA

When Shakti moves away from Shiva, everything in the universe is born, including the five elements that make up our entire material world. When an individual spirit (atman) is impelled to manifest a human form to work out the karma attached to it, individual Shakti (which is like a drop of water from the ocean of greater Shakti, and in Samkhya is known as prakriti), separates from Shiva at the crown of the head and moves down to the base of the spine, where it is held rooted in the body by an energetic force known as kundalini. Kundalini is the name given to the coil of energy that holds Shakti in human form. Traditionally, it is depicted as a sleeping green snake coiled three and a half times. The snake represents the grip of karma and spiritual ignorance (known as "greater *avidya*"), the essence of which is called the five *klesha*s. The five kleshas are:

1. *avidya:* ignorance of the true self. This klesha is one aspect of the greater avidya, which is the spiritual ignorance that results from all of the five kleshas.
2. *asmita:* ego. This is not the same as the Western idea of ego; here it is thought of as anything that separates us from truth and the divine, such as fear or hatred.
3. *raga:* attraction to things we like.
4. *dvesa:* repulsion toward things we don't like.
5. *abhinivesa:* fear of dying.

The kleshas are the limiting belief patterns of maya that cause us to remain ignorant of our own divinity.

The more you are trapped by avidya (comprising the five kleshas) and karma, the harder kundalini is to rouse. You want to awaken kundalini to remove the avidya that binds you to life in the material world and inhibits your awareness of the spiritual. When you awaken kundalini, you move toward enlightenment and a deeper understanding of all that is. When you learn how to release Shakti from the grip of avidya and karma, it can move back up the spine to reunite with Shiva at the crown of the head. With the union of Shakti and Shiva, you transcend the duality of the material world and return to a state of oneness to realize your true perfection. In order to stir kundalini and begin Shakti's ascent, it is important to practice asanas (the physical postures), *pranayama* (breath work), and meditation. These tools enable you to remerge your consciousness with that of the Divine Creator—the highest aim of Tantra.

During Shakti's initial journey away from Shiva and the birth of human form, atman directs prana to animate all of the elements (space, air, fire, water, and earth). The word *prana* means "vital life force": it animates life, matter, and mind. Without it, the elements could not hold together. Prana has five different qualities, called *vayus*, which animate each of the elements and give the lower five chakras their individual characteristics.

THE FIVE PRANA VAYUS

1. *apana:* Located in the genitals, anus, and lower extremities, apana regulates

the amount of earth in the body (through defecation, urination, menstrual flow, and ejaculation). Apana is also responsible for the evacuation of waste matter and toxins from every cell on exhalation (*langhana*).

2. *vyana:* Located all over the body, vyana enables circulation. It is related to the water element, as water circulates the nutrients of earth throughout the body.

3. *samana:* Located in the navel, samana is related to the fire element and regulates digestion and metabolism.

4. *prana:* Located in the chest and lungs, prana rides on the breath (air element) and is responsible for the absorption of life force on inhalation (*brahmana*).

5. *udana:* Located in the throat and related to space, udana draws energy upward to be used for speech and communication.

The prana vayus are best illustrated by a corpse. When someone dies, the first thing that happens is that the person ceases to communicate across space (udana). Then air (prana) leaves the body as the breath stops and all movement ceases. Without movement, fire (samana) dies and the body becomes cold. Finally, the body dries up and water (vyana) and earth (apana) separate. All of the elements return to their source. Without the five prana vayus, we would be nothing more than a sack of mixed-up elements!

All prana is distributed throughout the body by *nadis* (subtle channels of energy that control our physical, emotional, and spiritual health and well-being). The nadis are sometimes physically apparent (they include, for example, nerves and veins) but are mostly invisible to the naked eye; they are more often electromagnetic fields of energy. When the nadis are blocked, prana is prevented from moving freely in your system; your life force becomes sluggish, which can lead to ill health and disease.

We practice yoga to purify and reenergize the nadis and enable prana to flow freely. The ancient writings speak of 72,000 nadis. Of these, a few have special significance:

- *Sushumna nadi* runs from the base of the spine to the crown of the head, along the spinal cord, and when it is purified, Shakti can move up the spine to reunite with Shiva.

- *Ida nadi* runs from the left nostril to the midbrain, then coils through each chakra to the base of the spine and into the left side of the perineum. It is related to the parasympathetic nervous system and the more pacific, feminine energy of the moon.

- *Pingala nadi* runs from the right nostril to the midbrain, then coils through each chakra to the base of the spine and into the right side of the perineum. It is related to the sympathetic nervous system and the more dynamic, masculine energy of the sun.

THE SEVEN MAIN CHAKRAS

The seven main chakras (out of a total of 133 outlined in the yogic writings) that we will discuss in detail in this book run along the spine and are connected to sushumna nadi. In Sanskrit, *chakra* is the word for wheel. You can think of a chakra as a spinning concentration—a wheel of energy. You cannot actually see the chakras in your physical body, because they are fields of energy. The energy of each chakra corresponds to the physical, mental, and energetic aspects of the five elements that prana has brought to life, which constitute your being. The karmic content of all the chakras varies by individual and influences how they are experienced. The chakras are arranged vertically from the base of the spine to the crown of the head (see table 1).

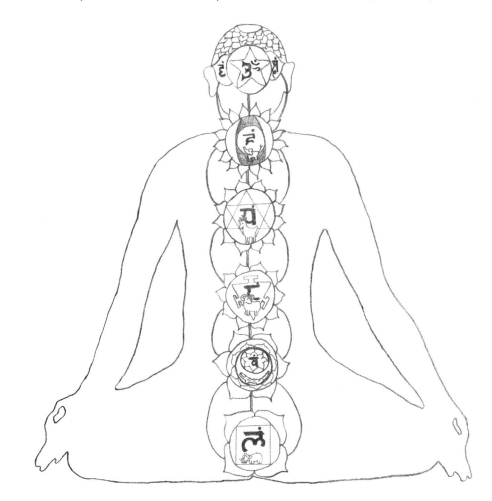

FIG. 1. *Chakras and Nadis.*

TABLE 1: THE CHAKRAS

Chakra	Location	Back-ground Color	Mantra	Yantra	Element (Bhuta)
MULADHARA	Pelvic floor, between pubis and tailbone	Red	LAM	Golden square	Earth
SVADHISHTHANA	Pelvic basin	Orange	VAM	Silver crescent moon, points touching	Water
MANIPURA	Solar plexus and navel	Yellow	RAM	Inverted red triangle	Fire
ANAHATA	Heart	Green	YAM	Blue six-pointed star	Air
VISHUDDHA	Throat	Blue	HAM	Smoky gray upward-pointing egg in a white circle	Space
AJNA	Third eye	Violet	KE-SHAM	Violet "eyelike" oval, tunnel of light with five beams	Command center of the elements
SAHASRARA	Crown	White	OM	Thousand-petaled lotus	Beyond the elements

Domain	Gland	Sense (Tanmatra)	Organ of Action (Karma indriya)	Organ of Knowledge (Jnana indriya)	Vayu
Material security; procreation instinct	Gonads	Smell: earth creates smell	Anus	Nose	Apana: energy of elimination
Sexuality; creativity; likes/dislikes; desire/lust; greed	Adrenals	Taste: water enables taste	Genitals	Tongue	Vyana: circulation
Introversion/extroversion; power/weakness	Pancreas	Sight: fire illuminates	Feet and legs	Eyes	Samana: heat and metabolism
Compassion; beginning of self-realization; sharing; unconditional love; selfless service; emotional clarity	Thymus	Touch: air enables touch	Hands	Skin	Prana: intake of energy
Wisdom; communication from higher mind	Thyroid	Sound: space provides medium for sound to travel	Vocal cords	Ears	Udana: communication
Full self-realization	Pituitary				
God-realization	Pineal				

The earth chakra, Muladhara, relates to the feet, legs, and pelvic floor, and through its solid constitution determines your relationship with the material world, matter, and form. Earth is the densest element, the base on which all the other elements rest.

The second chakra, Svadhishthana, is the water element that gives movement and enables the other elements to mix and form life. It is located in the pelvic basin and encompasses your reproductive organs. It relates to your sexuality and the realm of the unconscious mind.

The third chakra, Manipura, is governed by the element of fire. It is located around the navel and solar plexus. It relates to the heat in your body that is used for digestion and metabolism. Manipura chakra is responsible for your personal glow or radiance, as well as self-esteem.

These lower three chakras—Muladhara, Svadhishthana, and Manipura—are responsible for your self-image and how you relate to the world around you.

The fourth chakra, Anahata, is the center of the air element and resides in the chest and lungs. As clouds pass through the sky, this chakra, with its constant movement of the breath, is related to the changeable nature of your emotions.

Vishuddha, the fifth chakra, is the element of space and is located at the throat. It is your communication center. Vishuddha is related to space because sound must travel through space in order for you to communicate. This chakra is where you find your inner truth and communicate it to the world through personal expression.

Ajna chakra, situated in the midbrain, is the command center for the elements. Ajna allows us to see beyond the material world through the use of intuition, dreams, visualization, and imagination.

The seventh chakra, Sahasrara, is located at the crown of the head. It goes beyond the elements and is the part of us that transcends the material world. Sahasrara is where we reconnect with the divine force of Shiva through spiritual development and, ultimately, enlightenment.

In everyday life, the effects of the lower chakras become stored as feelings in Anahata. This influences your emotions, relationships with others, and ability to surrender. Anahata chakra is at the center of the chakra system and is responsible for integrating the lower and upper chakras, or the worlds of matter and spirit.

With the heart chakra as a linchpin, the higher chakras are concerned with developing our emotional and spiritual wisdom and enabling us to connect with our inner divinity to become inspired in our living.

The chakra system is symbolized by a lotus flower. The lotus has its roots in the mud, then the stem grows up through water, and finally above the water blossoms an incredible flower. The roots are down in the lower chakras and the stem grows up through water to the heart, the throat, and into the midbrain, which becomes the bud of the flower. Finally, the flower blossoms at the crown of the head. In darkness, the lotus flower closes to a bud and drops into the mud. When the sun rises, it blossoms. If we remain in darkness, then our lotus will never be able to blossom.

The chakras are where we receive, assimilate, and distribute our life energies. And through external situations (the pressures of life) or internal habits (poor physical alignment or self-destructiveness), a chakra can become imbalanced.

Like all phenomena, the chakras are broadly influenced by the three gunas: rajas (active), tamas (passive), and sattva (balanced). As I mentioned, the gunas are the principal forces of movement in nature and deal with the subtle energies behind all material and energetic phenomena.

When a chakra is rajasic, it is overactive and becomes a dominating force in a person's life. Conversely, an underactive, or tamasic, chakra is low in energy and thus has difficulty manifesting its energy in the world. In a sattvic state, a chakra is balanced. And when all of a person's chakras are sattvic, there is harmony and balance throughout.

The concepts of rajas, tamas, and sattva can be clearly illustrated in the fifth chakra, Vishuddha, located at the throat. This

chakra governs personal communication. When someone's Vishuddha chakra is rajasic, she will talk all the time and have trouble listening to what others have to say. This overactivity will be apparent in the neck and throat hyperextending over the torso, giving the impression that she is "in your face." In contrast, someone in whom Vishuddha chakra is tamasic will have difficulty with self-expression and shy away from communication. His neck and throat will retract into the torso, as if he is attempting to pull away from contact. A sattvic fifth chakra is seen in someone who is a relaxed, effective communicator.

The simplest way to balance each chakra is to create alignment in the physical body. Your body reflects your imbalances, acting as a mirror through which you can gauge how each chakra is functioning. When you align the body, you create balance, stability, and a solid base. This will make you more sensitive to the subtle qualities of the chakras, which you can then access through meditation.

Your asana practice is the first step toward aligning your body and balancing each chakra. Instead of changing the way the mind works to overcome years of patterns and beliefs—an extremely difficult and often superficial remedy—asana practice works to realign the physical energy centers that govern specific behaviors. I will teach you how to shape a physical yoga practice to suit your unique personality and circumstances. Once you have found balance in your body, I will then take you deeper with the meditation techniques in the online audio recording.

An understanding of the chakra system leads to an understanding of the self. The power to bring harmony and balance into your life will be within your grasp. The chakras are your doorways from the material world to the world of universal intelligence, intuition, and inspiration.

THE GUIDED MEDITATION PRACTICES

I have recorded a set of guided meditations to accompany the teachings in this book. You can access and download this audio recording at www.shambhala.com/chakra yoga.

The focus of these meditations is the chakras: the body's main physical, mental, and spiritual centers.

In the chakra meditations in the audio recording, I will guide you through a comprehensive chakra-balancing meditation. We start with a practice called Nadi Shodhana Pranayama, which is a breathing technique to balance the left and right sides of your brain. It enables you to draw your senses inward for meditation. We will then move through each chakra using a Bija mantra and a yantra to balance the energy of each chakra. Bija mantras are specific sounds that bring our awareness to the chakra and hold it there. Yantras are shapes that we visualize to balance the chakras' energy. Once we have moved through all the chakras, we will sit for eighteen minutes in silence to experience the state of oneness in which healing and universal love will flood every cell of your being. This meditation will be followed by a re-grounding practice and a closing mantra.

TWO

FINDING ROOTS

Muladhara, the Earth Chakra

HAVE YOU ever tried to stand on one leg? If you haven't, give it a try. When you only have half of your foundation, it's not very easy to find your balance, is it!

All living things need strong foundations. They cannot survive otherwise. Trees must have firm roots or they will fall in a storm. Animals must build their homes on safe ground. And humans, however mobile, still need a solid base in order to take the first steps toward higher consciousness. We are all—plants, animals, humans—connected to the world around us; the earth is the source of our sustenance and stability.

The base chakra, Muladhara, represents the earth, the densest of the five elements that make up life. We come from earth and to earth we return; it shapes all name (*nama*) and form (*rupa*) on the material plane.

Our origin, our identity, and our heritage are all seeds planted into Muladhara chakra at conception. These seeds take root, sprout, and shape our life. *Mula* translates as "root," "base," or "beginning," and *hara* as "the center." Muladhara is the base of our being and the center of our physical world.

Muladhara chakra is your source of power. When it is out of balance, this affects everything related to your personal stability and security. Muladhara controls how you deal with money, your body, and your family: your roots.

A few years ago I had a student who worked in the stock market. He was a very intelligent man and had lots of experience in his field. The only problem was that he kept losing money. He would invest at the right time and watch his investments grow, but when it came time to sell and take his profits, he was paralyzed. Time after time he would make money as the market gained momentum—then lose it again as the market fell. He had tried to overcome this problem by learning as much as possible about the stock market, talking to experts and reading every financial publication available, but nothing worked. He continued to lose money. He had all the intellectual knowledge he needed to be a success in the stock market, but he didn't trust his instincts enough to use his knowledge profitably. When he first came to see me and began doing yoga, things were so bad that he was worried he might lose his job.

I determined that he had an imbalance in Muladhara that was making it difficult for him to function decisively. We then worked together so that he could establish a firm foundation and change the habitual patterns that were limiting his growth. Today he gives the impression of someone who is confident and in control of his life, and he continues to grow through yoga and meditation.

Another one of my students who had an imbalance in Muladhara chakra had suffered for many years from compulsive eating and bulimia. No matter how many new therapies she tried, nothing seemed to help. When she came to see me, she had almost given up hope of ever being free of her disease. In fact, she had decided to try yoga because she thought it might help her to lose weight and curb her desire for food—she saw it as just another form of exercise. As Muladhara chakra is the center of those issues concerning how we treat and nourish our bodies, I began working with her physical structure in order to bring balance to her base. After a few months, we added meditation techniques to help her penetrate more deeply into the issues that were limiting her recovery. In addition to yoga, I recommended that she eat more whole, organic foods and drink an adequate amount of water. I also suggested that she minimize caffeine, sugar, and stimulants in order to purify her body and help it start to heal. Gradually, through yoga, meditation, and a balanced diet, she began to turn her life around. Her compulsiveness toward food decreased and finally vanished completely. Like everyone, she still has to deal with karma and the daily stresses of life; the difference now is that she comes to everything from a strong foundation.

Muladhara chakra is clearly related to questions of financial security and body image, but it can also involve issues relating to family. The chemical connection that is rooted into the first chakra is shared by both of our parents and our siblings as DNA. It links us on a deep, primal level. That is why we say "blood is thicker than water." Yet I like to joke that really it should be rephrased as "earth is denser than water." The genetic "earth" connection that exists in families transcends the emotional connection. We may argue with family members—we may even dislike them!—but we are still connected to them through the bond of Muladhara. If you have ongoing problems with your family and difficulty finding a resolution, balancing Muladhara will help. In order to determine whether you have an imbalance in Muladhara chakra, ask yourself the following questions:

- Does my life feel out of control?
- Do I find it difficult to make decisions?
- Do I suffer from financial insecurity?
- Do I act irresponsibly with regard to my money, my personal safety, or that of my family members?
- Do I feel poor, even though I have a solid bank account?
- Do I have an excessive concern for material wealth, to the point of being greedy?
- Do I find it difficult to nourish my body properly?
- Do I suffer from obesity, anorexia nervosa, or bulimia?
- Do I have ongoing problems with my parents, children, or other family members?

If you answered yes to any of these questions, working with Muladhara chakra will help you find equilibrium. Once you have achieved a stable foundation, you can tap into the inherent abundance of our planet and bring it into your life. You will be more comfortable with the possession of material wealth, without being possessed by it. You will be more comfortable with your place in the world and more content with what you have.

PHYSICAL LOCATION

Muladhara chakra is located at the base of the spine between the pubic bone, coccyx (tailbone), and ischial tuberosities (sitting bones). Its center is the perineum, which is

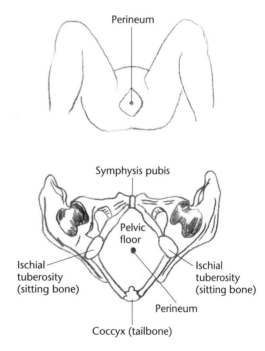

FIG. 2. *Pelvic floor and perineum.*

in the middle of the pelvic floor (also called the pelvic diaphragm) between the anus and genitals. The pelvic floor is the region below your pelvic cavity that keeps your internal organs in place.

The pelvic floor is influenced and affected by the muscles of the legs, and for this reason Muladhara chakra is also associated with the legs and feet. The integrity of the pelvic floor depends on the proper alignment of the legs and the balance of the feet, which act like the roots of a plant. We need our feet and legs to be firmly balanced in order to find grounding and stability.

If you stand on one leg when you are used to standing on two, then you can see how disorienting it is to be off balance. But even on two legs, the way we stand often creates imbalances in Muladhara chakra of which we may not be aware.

Think about your own life. Have you ever had days when you felt "rushed off your feet" or "a little off center"? We use these expressions without really thinking about their meaning, but they imply that Muladhara chakra is out of balance.

Just as the pelvic floor and the bones of the pelvis are intricately tied together, so are Muladhara and Svadhishthana chakras closely linked. The seeds of all action are in Muladhara, but they are fully expressed in Svadhishthana, which will be covered in the next chapter. Together, these chakras are the launch pad that gives the rocket of your spiritual awareness the support to move through the higher chakras and take off. If your launch pad is unstable, your rocket will never reach its destination.

In asana practice it is very important to bring Muladhara and Svadhishthana chakras into alignment: to build a solid life, you must start with a solid base. The following section explores the physical aspects of Muladhara chakra and will help you to determine your own imbalances, so that you can correct them. We will then expand upon these concepts to include the pelvic region of Svadhishthana in the next chapter. In teaching yoga, I always pay careful attention to the feet, legs, pelvic floor, and pelvis, in order to ensure that every pose has a solid foundation.

BALANCING YOUR FEET: CONNECTING TO EARTH

Standing correctly is the starting place for balancing Muladhara chakra. You must examine your feet carefully to determine how you stand and what you need to do in order to find stability. To find the usual position of your feet, jump up and down a few times and then examine the position of your feet after you land. Are they turning inward or outward? Is your weight more forward or backward? Do you have high or low arches? Do this a few times. Make a note of the way that you are most inclined to stand as we move on to the next exercise.

EXERCISE 1 FOOT STABILITY

To really feel how the position of your feet affects your balance, grab a partner for the following exercise.

Stand with your feet hip-distance apart and your toes turned in. **[A]** Have someone push on the middle of your chest. See how easy it is for you to be pushed off balance? Now stand with your feet hip-distance apart and your toes pointing outward. **[B]** Again have someone press on the center of your chest, and again see how easily you are pushed off balance. Now stand with your feet parallel and your weight evenly distributed on all four corners of your feet: base of big toe, inner heel, base of little toe, outer heel. **[C]** Try the exercise one last time. Notice that when your feet are stable and grounded, it is much easier to maintain your stability and balance.

Muladhara chakra is affected by many subtle alignments that begin with the feet: the position of your toes, how the weight is distributed between the balls and heels of your feet, the angle of your feet, the inner and outer arches of your feet, and the position of your heels in relationship to the broadest part of your feet (the span from the base of your big toes to the base of your little toes). All of these things must be in balance in order to set up a stable base, like a building's foundation, because the position of your feet affects your ankles, your calf and thigh muscles, your knees, and how the muscles of your legs interact with your hip structure and pelvic floor. This alignment affects your pelvis, torso, shoulder girdle, neck, and head. To maintain balance in your life, it is of the utmost importance to have your feet alive, vital, and in correct alignment. Once your feet are stable, you have the support to work upward.

EXERCISE 2 BLOCK EXERCISE

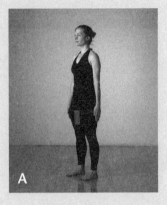

Observe your feet when you are standing. If you look down and your feet are pointing too far inward or outward, as in exercise 1, observe how this affects your legs (Are your knees knocking? Do you feel bowlegged? Are your thighs rotating inward or outward?), your pelvis (Does it tilt too far forward or backward?), your hips (Are both hip points pointing forward?), your torso (Is it centered over your pelvis and legs?), and your head (Is the crown of your head lengthening toward the sky?). As soon as you bring your feet back to parallel, you set your foundation. Then the inner and outer muscles of your legs work together to bring your ankles, knees, and hips in line, your pelvis comes into a neutral position, your spine lengthens, and your head floats comfortably on top of your shoulder girdle. The following exercise will help you to really feel this.

1. Place a yoga block (or a rolled towel) between your thighs. [A]

2. Make sure that your feet are parallel.

3. Push the block back, which will ro-

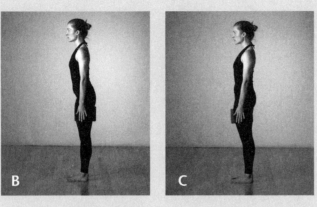

tate your thighs inward toward the wall be-hind you. **[B]** When this happens, feel how your tailbone and pubic bone move back, the inner arches of your feet drop down, and the outer arches of your feet lift up.

4. Now push the block forward, which will rotate your thighs outward. **[C]** Feel how your pubic bone moves up and your tailbone tucks under, and how your outer arch descends and your inner arch lifts up.

5. Repeat steps 3 and 4 a few times. Be careful not to let your knees lock, and try to feel the space—a light, open feeling—created in your ankle, knee, and hip joints.

6. Find the balance between the inner and outer rotation of your thighs. Feel the connection between your pubic bone and tailbone, the inner and outer rotations of your thighs, and the inner and outer arches of your feet: they all work together to create a stable foundation.

ASANAS

When you find the balance of Hatha yoga in Muladhara chakra, there is an amazing feeling of lightness and stability, as though you could stand forever! Muladhara is the foundation for the correct postural alignment yogis call Mountain Pose (Tadasana).

MOUNTAIN POSE
(Tadasana)

Mountain Pose is the foundation pose for all other yoga poses. When you understand the principles of alignment in Mountain Pose, you understand alignment in all of the other asanas. Mountain Pose brings the spine into a position that is optimal for maintaining its natural curves and is most efficient for bearing weight. It works with gravity so that the spine is supported by the vertebrae resting on top of each other.

Mountain Pose requires the least effort of all the standing poses, and it teaches proper alignment so as to prevent injury. The alignment in this pose also allows prana to flow freely, and it balances each of the different segments of the body and their related chakras. It may look easy from the outside, but feeling its internal dynamics requires sensitivity and awareness.

1. Bring your feet together with big toes touching, heels slightly apart, and check that your heel is lined up behind the broadest part of your foot (you may need to bring your feet slightly apart to get your

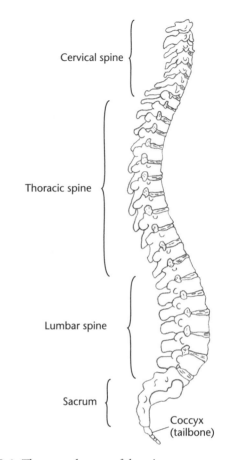

FIG. 3. *The natural curves of the spine.*

heel lined up correctly). Feel the four corners (ball of big toe, ball of little toe, inner and outer heel) of each foot anchored into the ground. Lift your toes, spread them wide, and lengthen them as you place them back down.

2. Find the balance between the inner and outer arches of your feet lifting and the inner and outer rotation of your thighs. Line up the crease between your second and third toes with the center of your knee and your hip joint. Feel your inner ankle bones

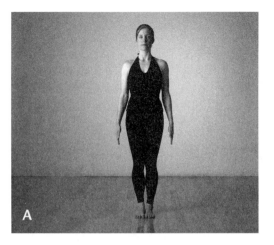 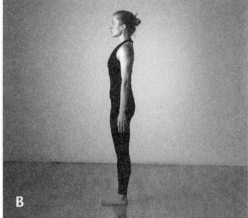

lift and separate. Broaden your calves and extend them down to your heels.

3. Feel your quadriceps muscles engage to lift your kneecaps toward your hips, but be sure not to hyperextend your knee. Feel the power in your feet and legs. Lift through your pelvic floor and lower belly while maintaining the natural curve of your lumbar spine.

4. Lift the front, back, and sides of your chest, but make sure your lower ribs are not poking forward.

5. Broaden across your breastbone and collarbones.

6. Relax your shoulders away from your ears as you feel your spine lengthen.

7. Let your head rest comfortably on top of your spine, without your chin tilting either too far up or too far down.

8. Relax your jaw and forehead.

9. Let your arms hang by your sides as if there were lead weights in your fingertips. [A]

10. Someone looking at you from the side in Mountain Pose should be able to draw a straight line through your ear, your shoulder joint, your hip joint, the center of your knee, and your anklebone. [B]

11. Breathe five deep, full breaths. Find both a softness and an inner strength.

Now we will go through a few asanas to illustrate how different movements of the body are affected by the actions of the feet, legs, and pelvic floor. We will apply the awareness of the previous exercises in a standing pose, forward bend, backward bend, inversion, and twist. Each pose will enhance your ability to feel Muladhara chakra in alignment.

1. WARRIOR POSE III
(Virabhadrasana III)

1. From Mountain Pose, extend your arms out to the side [A]. Take a medium step back with your left leg and come onto the ball of your left foot, keeping your hips squared forward.

2. Gently bend your right leg, and start to tilt your torso forward until your left leg lifts off the floor. Find length from the crown of your head to your heel, and try to maintain a sense of Mountain Pose in your body, as though you were standing upright (shoulders, hips, back [left] knee, and ankle in one line, back [left] foot flexed with all five toes pointing toward the floor). [B] Work to straighten your right leg as you keep your hips squared toward the floor. Eventually your arms, torso, and back leg are parallel to the floor and are supported by your standing leg, with each segment of your body still maintaining Mountain Pose alignment. [C]

3. As you tilt forward, keep lengthening through your lower back and feel the strength of your abdominal muscles working to hold you up. Let the back of your neck be long and keep your face relaxed.

4. If you are less strong, you can bring your hands onto your hips or onto blocks to support you. If you are stronger, you can extend your arms straight out in front of you.

5. Breathe five breaths.

6. Repeat on the other side.

Standing poses are very important for balancing Muladhara, because they safely de-

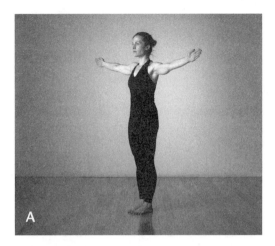

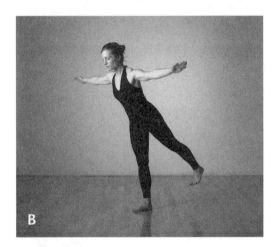

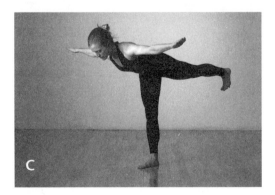

velop the strength of the legs and promote a strong foundation. When standing poses are done correctly, they balance and support the entire body. In Warrior Pose III you want to make sure that both legs are in Mountain Pose: your heel in line with the broadest part of your foot, the crease between your second and third toes in line with the center of your knee and hip joints, and all of the muscles of the legs working together as you lift through your pelvic floor. In this pose it is also very important that your hips are level and pointing straight forward, so that the muscles of the legs share the work equally. With a strong foundation, your abdominal muscles engage and strengthen your torso, and your back muscles work to bring length to your spine all the way up through the crown of your head.

2. STANDING FORWARD BEND (Uttanasana)

1. Take your feet hip-distance apart and check that the crease between your second and third toes, midknees, and hip joints are in line.

2. Balance your weight on all four corners of your feet.

3. Check that the inner and outer arches of your feet are equally lifted, your toes are spread wide, and there is a balance between the internal and external rotations of your thighs.

4. Bend your knees deeply and lower your hands to the floor in front and to the outsides of your feet.

5. Press down into all four points of the feet as you straighten your legs (make sure not to hyperextend your knees) and feel all of your leg muscles engage. Draw your shoulders up away from the floor and feel the back of your neck long and your head in a neutral position.

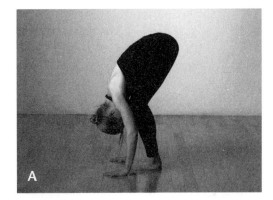

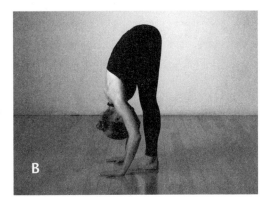

6. Breathe five deep breaths.

7. On each inhalation, feel a lifting of your chest and a lengthening of your spine.

8. On each exhalation, feel your belly draw in, which will allow you to bend forward more deeply.

9. Ride your breath as you would a wave in the ocean. Feel it raise you on each inhalation and release you on each exhalation. Once your feet, thighs, and sitting bones are in the right position, riding the breath will facilitate a graceful, deeper forward bend. Your pelvic floor will hold you up and keep you in a state of perfect balance.

In a forward bend, the inner and outer rotation of your thighs and the forward and backward movement of your legs set up a stable base for your pubic bone and tailbone to lift away from the floor and create length in your spine. Just as your feet have four corners, your legs have four sides: inside, outside, back, and front. You must balance all four corners of the feet and four sides of the legs in order to stabilize Muladhara chakra.

Standing Forward Bend really helps you to feel how the correct leg alignment creates a strong foundation. It is a very different feeling to do the forward bend with your weight too far forward in the balls of your feet, because then your quadriceps muscles become overly active. Similarly, if your weight is too far back in your heels, your hamstrings must work to hold you up. If your legs turn too far outward or inward, then your pelvis and pelvic floor shift and become imbalanced. Maintaining your stability in the forward bend will reinforce the balance in Muladhara chakra and help you to stay grounded in your life.

3. HIGH LUNGE
(Alana)

1. Start by kneeling on all fours.

2. Step your right foot up between your hands, [A] using blocks if you need to. [B]

3. Place your hands on the top of your right thigh and lift your torso to an upright position, so that your shoulders are in line with your hips. Lift your left knee up off the floor by tucking your toes under and pressing your heel away from you. [C] To modify the pose, keep your back knee on the floor.

4. Place your hands on your hips and square them so that both hips point forward. Align your left hip, knee, ankle, and foot to set up the inner and outer rotation of your left thigh. Make sure that your right knee is over your right ankle (so that your right leg forms a ninety-degree angle) and feel a balance between the inner and outer arches of your right foot.

5. Lower your arms beside you and feel how the solid foundation of your legs allows you to lift your chest away from your hips. Check that your torso is perpendicular to the floor. If your pelvis is tilting too far forward, bend your back knee to bring yourself upright. Engage the muscles of your pelvic floor and abdomen.

6. Bring both arms up into the air, with your hands shoulder-distance apart. Keep your shoulders away from your ears and your fingers pointed up toward the ceiling, palms facing each other. [D]

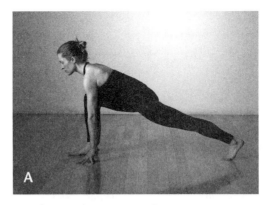

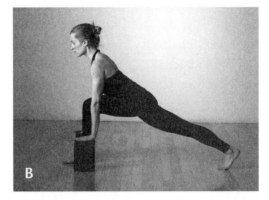

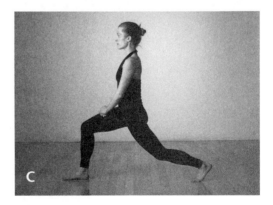

7. Feel your pelvic floor and abdominal muscles keep firming to hold you as you lengthen through your lower back. Open through your chest and feel how your thoracic spine slightly arches.

8. Breathe five deep breaths.

9. Repeat the entire exercise on the other side.

Finding the stability of Muladhara is of utmost importance to set up a base for back bending. High Lunge is the perfect pose to feel how the balance of your feet, legs, and pelvic floor interact to give you a stable base. It is important that the inner and outer rotations of your legs are balanced in back bending, so that your pelvis can be in the correct position for you to square your hips, firm your lower belly, and stabilize your lower back. If the hip flexor muscles of your back leg (psoas, quadriceps) are tight, it will tilt your pelvis too far forward (we will explore the pelvis more when we discuss Svadhishthana chakra in the next chapter), in which case you must keep your back leg slightly bent. You want your torso perpendicular to the floor so that you can lift and feel the back bend happening in the thoracic spine. This will avoid pinching and discomfort in the lower back.

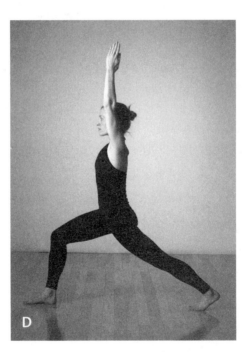

D

4. ENERGY REVERSAL POSE
(Viparita Karani)

1. Sit with one hip against a wall and your knees bent, feet flat on the floor.

2. Roll onto your side and then onto your back, lifting your legs up the wall as you do so. Your spine should now be at a right angle to your legs and the wall.

3. Your buttocks are against the wall and your lower back rests on the floor. (If you have tight hamstrings, bring your buttocks away from the wall so that you can straighten your legs without lifting your lower back.) Flex your feet, drawing back evenly through the big and little toes. Balance the inner and outer rotations of your legs and bring them parallel to each other and the wall. [A]

4. Feel your lower back lengthening and releasing and relax your abdominal muscles. Let your arms extend out to the sides at shoulder level, with your palms up. (If this creates tension in your neck or shoulders, you can rest your hands lower down by your sides.) Let your shoulders draw away from your ears, and keep the back of your neck long.

5. Slowly open your legs along the wall into a V, continually checking that the inner and outer rotations of your legs are balanced and that your feet are flexed at a right angle to the wall. [B] Notice how the rotation of your thighs influences the lifting of your pelvic floor. Feel how your pelvic floor acts as the center of gravity for the firming of your legs.

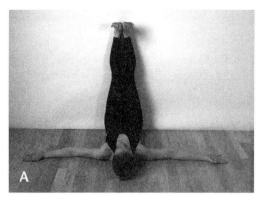

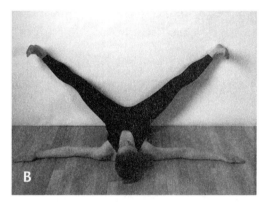

6. Try to hold the pose for up to two minutes, which will strengthen Muladhara chakra and take tension out of the backs of your legs and your inner thighs.

7. To come out of the pose, bring your hands to just behind and below your knees. Bend your knees and draw your legs together.

8. Roll over onto one side and slowly come up to a seated position.

When your legs and pelvic floor are active in an inversion, there is a sense of lightness and balance in the pose. You want to continually check that the big-toe and little-toe sides of your feet are drawing back evenly and that the inner and outer rotations of your thighs are balanced. Your hips, knees, and ankles should all be in line and your thighs firm, as though you were standing in Mountain Pose. The principles of alignment that you just used in Energy Reversal Pose will help you to balance Muladhara chakra in all other inverted poses in which your legs are in the air.

5. CROSS-LEGGED SPINAL TWIST
(Parivrtta Sukhasana)

We twist to the right first to compress the ascending colon, which moves up the right side of the body. We then twist to the left to compress the descending colon, which moves down the left side.

1. Sit in a modified cross-legged posture with both ankles on the floor and one heel in front of the other.

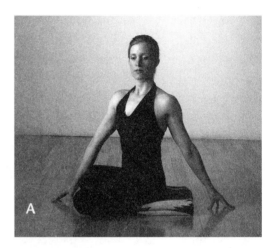

2. Lean forward and draw the flesh of your buttocks back and away so that you can sit comfortably balanced on the points of your sitting bones. (Do not draw your flesh back if you have a hamstring injury, to avoid exacerbating it.) If you need to, you can sit on a blanket to modify the pose. **[A]**

3. Sit up tall and balance the inner and outer rotations of your thighs to stabilize your base. Check that your hips are squared forward.

4. Bring your fingertips onto the floor in front of you.

5. Inhale and raise your right arm into the air. Lengthen your spine.

6. Exhale and lower your right arm to the floor behind you. **[B]** Feel your lower

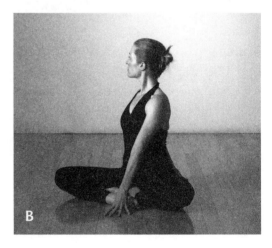

abdomen moving toward your right hip as you try to keep your hip structure stable. Move the twist up through your thoracic (middle) spine and then let your head follow gracefully.

7. On each inhalation, feel your spine lengthen and your body expand. On each exhalation, move deeper into the space that your inhalation has created. Repeat this process as you breathe and deepen into the twist.

8. Come back to center and repeat the twist to the left.

It is important to keep both of your sitting bones firmly rooted into the floor and your hips pointing forward in order to stabilize your pelvis. In seated poses your sitting bones become like feet, so you want to make sure that you are not sitting too far back or too far forward. Once you have secured your base and feel a lifting through your pelvic floor, you have set the foundation in Muladhara chakra. From there, feel your abdominal muscles engaged and a lengthening through your spine as you come into the twist. As in this Cross-Legged Spinal Twist, all twisting requires a stable base so that the twist can happen in the thoracic spine and up through the shoulder girdle. You want to avoid leading the twist with the neck and shoulders, or twisting in the lumbar spine, which has only five degrees of rotation.

THREE

DISCOVERING FLOW

Svadhishthana, the Water Chakra

THE SECOND CHAKRA, Svadhish-thana, means "the favored place" or "the place of *sva*," the place of self. The qualities of Svadhishthana are *ragas* (attraction) and *dvesa* (repulsion); they are your likes and dislikes—in a word, taste. Svadhishthana chakra also acts as the storehouse of your unconscious mind and governs your impulses and desires. This chakra is about the need to take action. It is where you set your *sam kalpha,* your intention.

To explain the unconscious in Svadhish-thana, I like to use the analogy of a parrot. You can teach a parrot to say, "Good morning, you look great!" You can teach it to say, "Wow, you're a genius!" But if you open the cage and take it by the neck, it won't say, "Please let me go"; it will squawk and try to bite you. Its true nature will come out.

Svadhishthana is associated with the element of water, which is the second-densest element. Water brings movement to the other elements and mixes them together to create life. Without water, life could not exist.

The water element links us to the tides. As the tides flow in and out, so much of our life is spent pushing away what we don't like and trying to attract more of what we do. We think that if we get everything we want it will bring us happiness, yet once we've achieved whatever it is we think will make us happy, we go on to look for something else.

Haven't you noticed that when you really want something, you'll put a huge amount of effort into getting it—even if it's just a pair of shoes? You save your money, go to a number of different shoe stores, and finally select your purchase. But then once you have the shoes in the bag, you start to think about another pair in a different color, or a matching belt. Immediately your mind starts searching anew, because it is never satisfied.

We strive to find happiness through our senses, yet our desires can be only temporarily fulfilled. Satisfaction is fleeting. When Svadhishthana chakra is out of balance, we spend all our time rejecting what we don't like and embracing what we do.

Water holds enormous power. When it is stored and directed, it can do all sorts of things, from making electricity to grinding corn. But if it is dispersed, it loses its potency. If you can learn to effectively harness and channel your water element in Svadhishthana chakra, you can overcome the patterns of your unconscious mind and find greater fulfillment in life.

I had a student who had tried for years to quit smoking. Every New Year's Day he would say to himself, "I'm going to give up smoking," but by the end of the day his resolution had, well, gone up in smoke. He had the best conscious intentions, but as soon as something unpleasant or annoying occurred, his unconscious would take over. On the one hand he was thinking, "I shouldn't smoke. It's terrible. It's cancerous, and I should quit." On the other hand, after a quarrel with his wife, he would take out his cigarettes and say, "I like smoking. Why should I bother quitting? Who cares if I die? Anyway, I can always try to quit again next year"—and he would light up again. Svadhishthana chakra was what really governed him; to make changes, he had to purify it. Using the same tools that I outline in this book, we worked physically and energetically to balance Svadhishthana chakra and break the unconscious patterns of his mind. Three years ago he quit smoking for good.

Another student had trouble with personal relationships. Instead of enjoying a long-term commitment, she had a series of brief affairs and one-night stands. She would meet someone, fall in love for a day, a week, or a month, and then find that the person was not as appealing as she thought and start looking for the next perfect thing. She wanted rapture and went from person to person to maintain the high. However, because no relationship had promise or meaning, she would quickly become bored and frustrated with her partner and move on. When she first came to see me, she told me that what she really wanted was to settle down and start a family. I spent time working with her to overcome the unconscious patterns that were driving her life, and after a few months of yoga and meditation she began to break her destructive habits. A year later she met a wonderful man and was able to work with him over time to establish a loving relationship. Although this woman, like everyone, still has her weaknesses and vulnerabilities, she has uncovered a deeper contentment within that has helped her to establish and maintain a committed relationship.

When Svadhishthana chakra is out of balance, nothing and no one is ever enough. Life has no constancy. You feel fragmented and volatile. Your desires dominate and oblige you to seek satisfaction through the senses: sex, food, material possessions, status. To determine whether you have an imbalance in Svadhishthana chakra, ask yourself the following questions:

• Do I have difficulty sustaining relationships?
• Am I compulsive?
• Do I suffer from an overabundance or lack of desire?
• Do I make resolutions (for example, to quit smoking) without the power to carry them out?
• Do I become addicted easily?

If you answer yes to any of these questions, balancing Svadhishthana chakra will help you transcend the sensual world and truly come into the oneness of yoga. Working in Svadhishthana, you can go beyond the frustrations of material desire to become whole again.

PHYSICAL LOCATION

Svadhishthana is located in the pelvic basin between the anterior superior iliac spine (ASIS) and the ischial tuberosities (sitting bones). It is in the bowl of the pelvis, right in front of the sacrum.

You must obtain a balanced relationship between the ASIS and the sitting bones in order to regulate the position of the pelvis

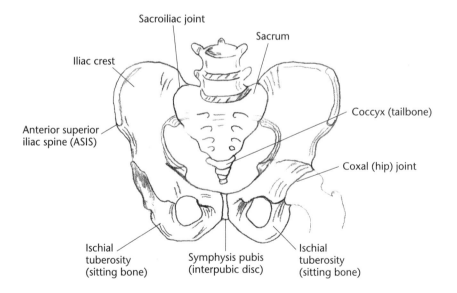

FIG. 4. *Pelvis and hip structure.*

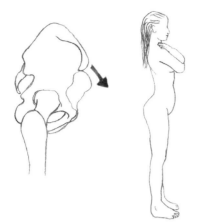

FIG. 5. *Pelvis tilting forward.*

and find balance in Svadhishthana chakra. If the muscles that pull the ASIS forward (psoas, quadriceps) are too tight and/or the muscles that draw the sitting bones down (hamstrings) are too weak, the pelvis will tilt too far forward, the muscles of the abdomen will become flaccid, and the lumbar curve will become more pronounced. (We will discuss the ramifications of this in the next chapter.) Someone whose pelvis is tilted forward will be overactive in this chakra (for example, sexually compulsive).

EXERCISE 1 CHAIR POSE (Utkatasana)

One of the best poses for experiencing the activity of the pelvis is Chair Pose (Utkatasana). When you practice this pose, you need to project your sitting bones back in order to sit down, but if you don't lift the ASIS up in the front, you will feel pressure and strain in your lower back.

1. Starting with your feet hip-distance apart and your hands on your thighs, bend your knees slightly as if attempting to sit down on a chair. Keep your heels on the floor and your knees tracking directly over your toes.

2. Let your spine rise up out of your hips, which will create the sensation of a firming in the lower belly. Be careful not to stick your seat out too much, or you will overly arch your spine. [A] Also try not to draw your sitting bones too far under, which will cause you to round in the middle of your back. [B]

3. Place your fingers on the pointy protuberances at the front of your hip bones (these are your ASIS) and tilt your pelvis forward and back a few times. Try to find a balance between the two.

4. Once you feel as if you have found

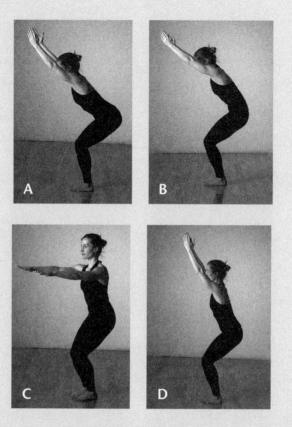

the balance in your pelvis, keep your breastbone lifted and breathe deeply for five breaths. Lift your arms straight out in front of you with your palms down and parallel to the floor. **[C]** If you have tight shoulders, stay in this position. If you are more open, slowly extend your arms upward as you try to keep your shoulders from lifting up toward your ears. **[D]**

5. Inhale as you slowly stand up. Relax your arms alongside your body.

As you become aware of how your pelvis interacts with the rest of your body, you can apply these principles throughout your asana practice. Seek to find the balance between the lifting-up through the ASIS in front and the drawing-back of the sitting bones. This will help you to find lightness and balance in Svadhishthana chakra.

EXERCISE 2 TANTRIC HAND GAZING

Muladhara chakra governs the instinct for procreation, but Svadhishthana chakra is where we express our sexual urges. Stabilizing Svadhishthana chakra is critical to regulating sexual activity and developing good relationships. As I mentioned in the previous chapter, it is important to understand that Muladhara and Svadhishthana chakra work together; the sexual instincts that are grounded in Muladhara find expression in Svadhishthana. This is shown physically in the way the pelvic floor (Muladhara) acts as a foundation for the pelvis and genitals (Svadhishthana).

In Tantra, a perfect balance between male and female energies is sought in sexual union. This is not to imply that sex should be limited to a male and a female, because in homosexual relationships one partner will have more male or more female energy. To get a sense of the way sexual energy is looked at in Tantra, take a few minutes to do the following exercise.

1. Look at your hand.
2. Now close your eyes and look at your hand as if from the inside. Try to really feel the bones, muscles, and tendons under your skin.
3. Again, look at your hand, but feel it from the inside as well.

Looking at the hand and feeling it simultaneously is the tantric way. It is more than just seeing the exterior. When you limit perception to your eyes, you may notice that your hands are dry, that your fingernails are rough, or that you have the same hands as your mother, but when you feel your hand from the inside as well as seeing it, you add another dimension—a glow, a presence—to your awareness.

Similarly, if we look at sex only through the lens of the senses, we get a very superficial view. But to feel and experience from the inside is to truly appreciate the sexual union of male and female. When these two opposite forces unite, the energy of Shakti begins to move. Sex becomes a spiritual exercise that culminates in Shakti's reunion with Shiva.

Although the roots of sexuality are in the two base chakras, sexual energy exists in every chakra. As we already discussed, the second chakra is concerned with attraction and repulsion, while the third chakra governs all of our ego needs concerning sex. The fourth chakra influences all of the associated sexual emotions, positive and negative, while the fifth chakra deals with our ability to communicate our sexual needs and feelings. Ultimately, spiritual sex leads to the union of Shiva and Shakti in

Ajna, the sixth chakra. And in the seventh chakra, Sahasrara, we go beyond temporal sex to merge with the energy of the divine.

Sex really can transcend the physical act of intercourse. When two people have bonded, merely touching and holding—even exchanging a look—can be enough to maintain a strong connection. When we unite with another person to experience a life together, we grow toward spiritual consciousness.

From a tantric perspective, when sexual energy is diverted upward through the chakras instead of outward through the physical release of orgasm, it is a divine experience. The feeling that we get when Shakti moves to Shiva is the same feeling of release that we experience during orgasm, only more powerful. It becomes another path to bliss, akin to meditation.

If the muscles of the lower abdomen are tight and/or there is a shortness or tightness in the hamstrings, then the sitting bones will be pulled too far down and the pelvis will tilt backward, flattening out the lumbar curve. In this case, energy in Svadhishthana chakra will be directed more inward (creating a lack of desire).

In order to find lightness and energy in Svadhishthana chakra, you must balance your pelvis. When this happens, you can effectively channel its power to break the unconscious patterns in your life.

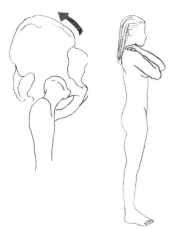

FIG. 6. *Pelvis tilting backward.*

ASANAS

Now we will go through a few asanas to illustrate how different movements of the body are affected by the actions of the pelvis. We will apply the awareness of the previous exercises in a standing pose, forward bend, backward bend, inversion, and twist. Each pose will enhance your ability to feel Svadhishthana chakra in alignment.

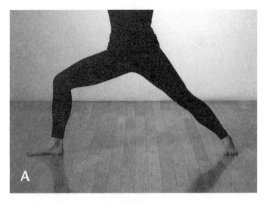

1. WARRIOR POSE II
(**Virabhadrasana II**)

1. From Mountain Pose, step your left foot back four feet and place it parallel to the back edge of your mat. Check that your right foot is parallel to the outer edges of your mat. A line drawn from the heel of your right foot should intersect your left arch. **[A]**

2. Check that your hip bones are level. If your hips are tight, you can let your left hip rotate forward and your left foot turn in a little. In this position your hips will turn slightly toward your front leg, instead of squaring to the side. **[B]** Keep your left foot, knee, and hip in line with each other.

3. Bend your right knee so that it is directly over your right ankle. Aim to get your right thigh parallel to the floor. You may need to widen or narrow your stance to keep your right leg bent at a ninety-degree angle and your right knee pointing forward.

4. Feel your pelvic floor and abdomen engaged, the weight of your torso centered

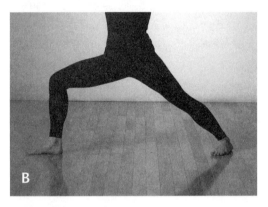

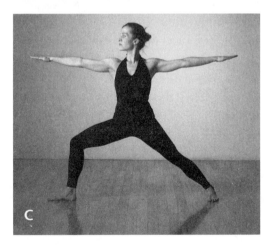

between your legs, and your rib cage centered directly over your pelvis. Your pelvis is in a neutral position and both of your ASIS are level. (We have two anterior superior iliac spines, both of which must be squared and level.)

5. Position your shoulders directly above your hips so that your torso is perpendicular to the floor. Try to keep your torso facing sideways and your spine long.

6. Hold your arms out at shoulder level, parallel to the floor and stretching toward either end of the mat. Your shoulders should stay relaxed and away from your ears, and your fingers should be together. [C]

7. Feel your feet drawing together (although they will not actually move) to engage the muscles of your legs and set up a lifting through your pelvic floor.

8. Let your eyes gaze out past the middle finger of the right hand.

Coming out of the pose:

9. Straighten your right leg and lower your arms alongside your body.

10. Realign your feet and repeat the pose on the other side.

Warrior Pose II strengthens your legs and brings greater awareness of how your legs interact with and stabilize your pelvis. It is important to position your feet at the proper angle: front foot parallel to the outer edges of your mat and back foot parallel to the back of the mat or slightly turned in, depending on the openness in your hips. With your feet in that position, your foundation has been set. Then you can firm the thighs and concentrate on the correct inward and outward rotations of the legs (front thigh rotates out, back leg rotates in). This will set your pelvis in a neutral position so that your spine can project upward and perpendicular to the floor. When your pelvis is correctly positioned in Warrior II, you will be able to engage your lower abdomen and find spaciousness and strength in the natural curve of your lumbar spine, as well as lengthening through the sides of your body and up through the crown of your head.

2. SEATED WIDE ANGLE POSE
(Upavista Konasana)

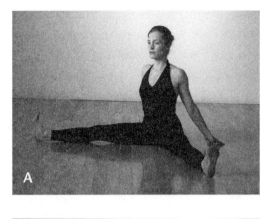

1. Sit on the floor with your spine tall and your legs spread apart as wide as is comfortable. (If you are very flexible, do not open your legs too wide or you will overstretch the ligaments in your hips.)

2. Make sure that the second toe crease, knee, and hip of each leg are in line and that your feet are flexed (press out through all four corners of your feet). Feel the inner and outer arches of your feet lift, your toes spread wide, and your quadriceps engaged. Balance the inner and outer rotations of your legs and check that your toes and knees point straight up. Do not hyperextend your knees.

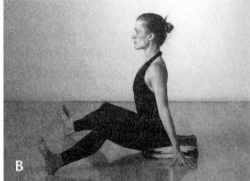

3. Draw the fleshy part of your seat back and bring your fingertips onto the floor behind you. Balance your weight evenly on your sitting bones, engage your pelvic floor and abdomen, and lengthen the crown of your head toward the ceiling. **[A]**

4. If you are tight and find that your pelvis is tilting back (your spine stays rounded when you try to sit tall), sit on a blanket and bend your knees. **[B]**

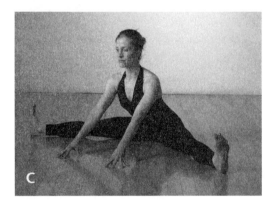

5. Bend forward from your pelvis and bring your arms in front of you as you lead your breastbone forward between your legs. Keep your head in line with the rest of your spine to prevent your chin from jutting forward, and relax your shoulders away from your ears. **[C]**

Seated Wide Angle Pose helps to find the balance in Svadhishthana chakra, because you can feel how the position of your pelvis influences your ability to find Mountain Pose (Tadasana) in the rest of your body. On the one hand, if your hamstrings are tight, your pelvis will tilt too far back, your legs will roll outward, your spine will round, and you will be unable to lengthen forward. **[D]** If this is the case, you can sit on a blanket or keep your knees bent. On the other hand, if you tilt too far forward, your thighs will roll in, you will overarch through your spine, and the back of your neck will be compressed. **[E]** In Seated Wide Angle Pose the pelvis is the fulcrum of the pose and needs to be in a neutral position to balance Svadhishthana chakra.

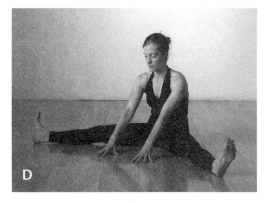

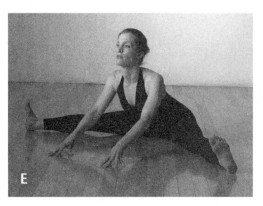

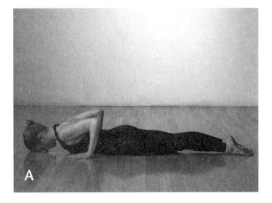
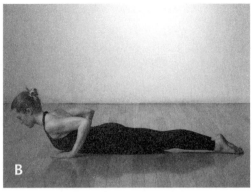

3. COBRA POSE
(Bhujangasana)

1. Lying face down on your belly, place your hands flat on the floor underneath your shoulders and your elbows near the sides of your body and pointing back toward your hips.

2. Rest the tops of your feet on the floor with your toes pointing away from you. Press all ten toenails into the floor. Check that your legs are in Mountain Pose, parallel, and engaged (most people need to rotate the thighs inward to find Mountain Pose in this position). Your feet are either hip-distance apart or together (which is harder). Press your pubic bone down into the floor and engage your pelvic floor and abdominal muscles. Feel your lower back lengthening. Be careful not to grip your buttocks. **[A]**

3. Inhale, lift your chest off the floor, and lengthen it forward. Feel your shoulder blades sliding down your back as you continue to lengthen your spine. **[B]**

4. Draw your legs back and away from your breastbone as it moves forward. Keep engaging your abdominal muscles and thinking about rotating your legs inward to maintain length and openness through your lower back. Feel the back bend in your thoracic spine. Use your back muscles, not your arm strength, to lift your upper torso comfortably away from the floor.

5. Keep your pubic bone pressing into the floor; try not to rest on your belly.

6. Hold the pose for five breaths.

In Cobra Pose you do not want to feel any pressure in your lumbar spine. Internally rotating the legs widens the lower back and creates space so that you can then lengthen your tailbone down toward your heels. This action balances Svadhishthana chakra and supports the back bend in your thoracic spine.

4. DOWNWARD-FACING DOG POSE
(Adho Mukha Svanasana)

1. Begin on all fours with your hands slightly forward of your shoulders and your knees under or slightly behind your hips (depending on how much space you need between your hands and feet in order to get the maximum length in your spine when you come into Downdog).

2. Spread your fingers comfortably wide. Make sure that your middle fingers are pointing forward and parallel to each other.

3. Curl your toes under, press the pads of your toes into the mat, and press your hands firmly into the floor. **[A]**

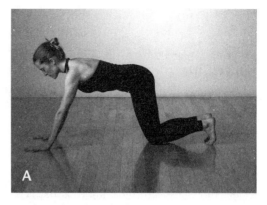

4. Contract your thighs to lift your knees off the floor. Move your hips back over your heels and then lift your hips up toward the ceiling as you straighten your legs.

5. Try to create an upside-down V with your body as you lengthen down through the backs of your legs and your spine. If you are tight, you can keep your knees bent to prevent your pelvis tilting back and rounding in your spine. **[B]**

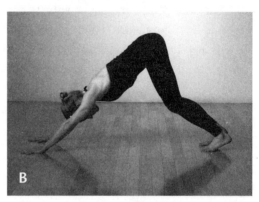

6. Inhale and feel all of the muscles of your legs engage, turn your sitting bones up to the sky (if you are very flexible, make sure your pelvis does not overrotate and cause too much arching through your spine), and press your heels to the floor. Check that your legs are in Mountain Pose (your heels should be hidden behind the widest part of your foot). **[C]**

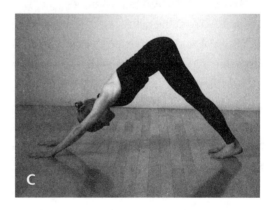

7. Press firmly into your thumbs and forefingers and lift up out of your wrists; feel your forearms turn in slightly. At the same time, externally rotate your upper arm bones (i.e., turn the wrinkly part of your elbow toward the floor) outward and draw your shoulders away from your ears. Keep your elbows straight but not locked.

8. Feel the weight evenly distributed between your arms and legs. Relax your face and head. Gently nod and shake your head "yes" and "no" to ensure that you are not holding any tension in your neck. Relax your jaw. Your gaze should be toward your feet with the back of your neck long.

9. Keep lengthening your spine.

10. Take five deep breaths.

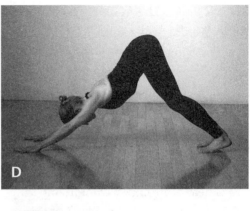

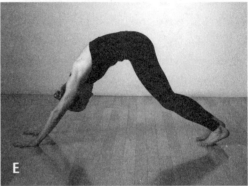

Downward-Facing Dog is a great pose for exploring proper alignment. In Downward-Facing Dog, the pelvis plays a major role. In a supple person, the pelvis is liable to tilt too far forward and create excessive arching in the spine. [D] In someone with tight hamstrings, the sitting bones draw down, which may pull the pelvis back and cause rounding through the spine. [E] (If this is happening to you, keep your knees bent.) You are trying to keep the natural curves of the spine and find space between each vertebra. This will bring a feeling of lightness to your pelvis and a balance to Svadhishthana chakra.

5. MALTESE TWIST
(Jathara Parivartanasana)

We twist to the right first to compress the ascending colon, which moves up the right side of the body. We then twist to the left to compress the descending colon, which moves down the left side.

1. Lie on your back with your legs together and knees bent and your feet flat on the floor. Extend your arms out to your sides in line with your shoulders, palms up. **[A]**

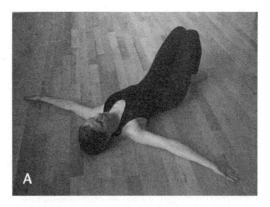

2. Lift your seat two inches off the floor, shift your hips to the left three to four inches, and place them back down. **[B]**

3. Keeping your back where it is, draw your knees to your chest and then drop them over to the right (opposite the side to which you shifted your hips in step 2). **[C]** This aligns your spine correctly for the twist.

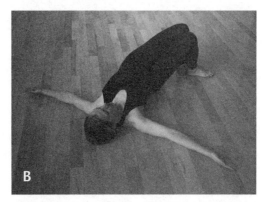

4. Your spine should be in one line from the crown of your head down to your tailbone, and your hips and knees stacked one on top of the other. Your gaze should be toward the ceiling. Or, if it is comfortable for your neck, you can gaze over your left shoulder. Your thighs should be at a ninety-degree angle to your torso and your lower legs at a ninety-degree angle to your thighs.

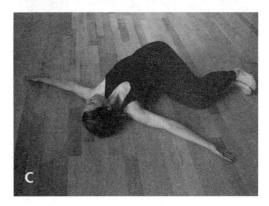

5. Check to make sure that your knees stay together. Use your right hand to hold on to your left knee and keep it correctly aligned. This keeps your pelvis and hip structure stable. Let your left arm extend

out to the side as you keep your shoulders relaxing away from your ears. Do not worry if your left shoulder comes off the floor.

6. Take five deep breaths.

7. Repeat the same sequence on the other side.

In Maltese Twist you must bring your pelvis into a neutral position to find the necessary relationship between your ASIS and sitting bones to balance Svadhishthana chakra. This sets up a firm foundation so that the twist can happen in the thoracic spine.

FOUR

ILLUMINATING GEMS

Manipura, the Fire Chakra

MANIPURA IS the home of your fire element and literally means "city of gems." When you have the right balance of fire in Manipura, it is like shining a light on a treasure chest overflowing with gems—every cell of your being is filled with brilliance!

The fire in Manipura chakra gives you your "glow," burnishes your ego, and illuminates your mind; it helps you to see the world around you clearly. This fire also creates the necessary heat for the metabolism of food, cellular transactions, and thought.

If the fire in Manipura chakra blazes out of control, it can blind you to your own faults, leading to egotism. People with too much fire have a fierce intelligence but can come across as arrogant, vain, and insensitive. They believe they are always right,

get angry easily, and seek to control others through their anger. If the fire in Manipura is inadequate, it makes you depressed, insecure, and extremely introverted; it becomes hard to see your life clearly, leading to a feeling of heightened vulnerability.

In order to determine whether you have an imbalance in Manipura chakra, ask yourself the following questions:

- Do I have trouble making decisions?
- Do I feel nervous in group situations and prefer to spend most of my time alone?
- Do I suffer from low self-esteem? Constant self-doubt?
- Do I engage in self-destructive behavior?
- Am I always right, whatever the argument?

- Have I been accused of insensitivity or intolerance?
- Do I have a hard time working with others?

Balancing Manipura chakra will correct personality problems and promote an equitable approach to yourself and others. Your ego will no longer need continual gratification. You will discover a moderation in thought and action. I call this "obtaining perspective of the ego": you are able to listen to people without being overwhelmed by them. You instinctively find a comfortable relationship with the world. Your character becomes gemlike: solid, multifaceted, filled with light.

It is easy to notice when someone's fire is unsteady. Many years ago I had a student whose fire was weak; her gems had lost their luster. When I first started teaching her she was depressed, introverted, and lacking a healthy ego; in class she always set up her mat at the back of the room and tried to make herself invisible. When I approached to help her with her postures, she would apologize, as if she wasn't worth the attention. Her fire in Manipura was almost extinguished.

After a few years of yoga practice, with a more stable and balanced Manipura chakra, she asked to meet me privately after class. She confided to me that yoga had greatly improved her self-esteem and her inner vision. When she first started practicing yoga, she had fallen into a series of destructive relationships with men who used and discarded her. She had felt powerless to exert control over her life. Now, she said, she was in charge again. She no longer wanted to hurt herself. She was free.

Finding the right amount of fire in Manipura enabled my student to study herself and the effects of her actions objectively. By turning inward she discovered and recognized the valuable treasure within, which gave her the strength to act in her best interests and break the cycle of harmful relationships. Today, after practicing for six years, she has changed considerably—at ease in class and happy to ask questions about her practice in front of the whole group. She is in a healthy relationship and recently began her training as a teacher of yoga, eager to bring others the joy she has found.

Contrast her case with another of my students who had too much fire. He would come into class with a swagger, place his mat at the front, and take up more of my time and energy than anyone else. He was so demanding and arrogant that other students—and staff—complained to me about him. I wasn't surprised when he took me aside after a few months of practice and asked for my advice. He owned a small business, which required him to manage people and delegate responsibility, but he couldn't trust his staff to do the work properly and ended up doing it all himself. It soon became clear that he was very harsh and critical of his employees, which led to low morale and a high turnover. His internal fire blinded him to how he had created an environment where his staff had no room for self-expression, no job satisfaction, and no company loyalty. He was so overloaded with work that he was in danger of a complete collapse.

My student needed to get his fire under control so that he could observe himself and see how his behavior affected others. He had to learn how to share power in order to become a successful manager of people. I gave him some exercises to contain his fire, and gradually his gems went from blazing wildly to sparkling softly. Recently he told me that he had started to listen to his employees and that their advice was helping him to make improvements in his business.

PHYSICAL LOCATION

Manipura is located in the lower torso and runs from the pubic line to the xiphoid process at the base of the sternum. It encompasses the abdominal wall (rectus abdominis, transversus abdominis, and internal and external obliques), lumbar fasciae, psoas, quadratus lumborum, and erector spinae muscles of the lower back, which surround the five vertebrae that make up the lumbar curve.

The concentration of heat in Manipura chakra developed as human beings evolved into bipeds and the curves of the spine emerged; these muscles had to be strong in order to lift and hold us upright and to provide the refined heat needed to fuel our processes of higher thought. Quadrupeds don't have the same broad muscles that

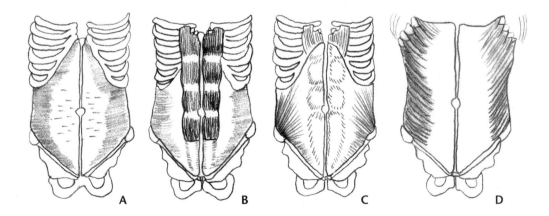

FIG. 7. *Abdominal wall: (A) transversus abdominis, (B) rectus abdominis, (C) internal oblique, (D) external oblique*

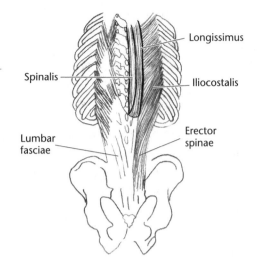

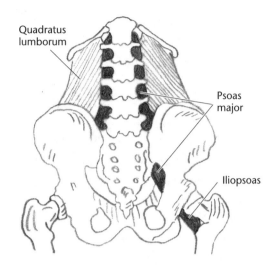

FIG. 8A. *Lumbar fasciae and erector spinae.*

FIG. 8B. *Posterior view of abdominal wall muscles.*

we do in this area; if you have a dog, feel its lower back—there is hardly any muscle there.

If the muscles of the rectus abdominis, the erector spinae, and the psoas are not in balance, this affects the lumbar curvature of the spine. When the lumbar curve is too pronounced, it is called lordosis. This causes the heat of the body to radiate outward, which goes hand in hand with overly aggressive and domineering behavior.

In the opposite case, when the lumbar

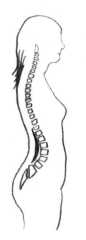

FIG. 9. *Lordosis.*

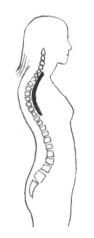

FIG. 10. *Torso caved in (thoracic kyphosis).*

EXERCISE 1 TANTRIC WALKING

Learning to walk properly brings Manipura chakra into balance and gives you the right amount of fire to move efficiently through life. Walking correctly also balances the other chakras, because each chakra corresponds to a specific part of your foot. The bone of your heel corresponds to Muladhara chakra and is your solid base. The outside flesh of the heel links to Svadhishthana chakra, which is motivation and movement. Manipura chakra is the outer arch of the foot, related to the lumbar curve. Anahata chakra is the ball of the foot, which lifts you as you move through the air. Vishuddha chakra is in the toes that launch you forward into space. The position of your feet when you walk affects the way energy moves in your body. In order for you to balance the chakras, with each step you must first feel the heel of your foot connect to the floor, then the outside of the heel into the outer arch. Finally, the weight transfers to the ball of your foot and you spring off your toes before starting the whole process again on the other side. This way of walking moves the energy through the chakras from the base upward and brings a lightness that travels from your feet all the way up through the crown of your head.

1. Find a straight line on the floor.

2. Begin to walk forward, placing your feet on either side of the line

3. With each step, feel the heel of the foot connect to the floor and then roll to the outer arch, the ball of the foot, and finally spring off the toes.

EXERCISE 2 INCLINE PLANK POSE
(Ardha Chaturanga Dandasana)

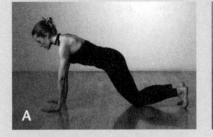

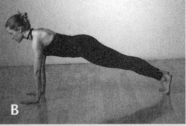

1. Begin by kneeling on all fours. Then lift your knees off the floor and straighten your legs as if you were about to do a push-up. If you cannot lift up your body weight, keep your knees on the floor to modify the pose. **[A]** Bring your wrists and elbows directly underneath your shoulders. Do not lock your elbows.

2. Feel your abdominal muscles and pelvic floor firming to help keep your hips from sinking down, but do not let your seat lift too high. You want your pelvis in a neutral position. If your knees are off the floor, press your heels backward and feel all of your leg muscles engage and your inner thighs lift up, maintaining a straight line from the crown of your head to your ankles. **[B]** Feel your weight evenly distributed between your hands and feet. If your knees are on the floor, let your hips lower so that you have a straight line from your knees to your armpits.

3. Draw your shoulder blades toward each other and slightly down your back as you feel your spine lengthen. The alignment in this pose is the same as Mountain Pose, except that you are facing the floor.

Incline Plank Pose is an excellent pose for strengthening the entire body and feeling how the abdominal and back muscles must work in tandem to hold you up. If your abdominal and back muscles are weak, you will have a hard time keeping your hips lifted (causing your belly to fall toward the floor and your back to arch), or you will lift your hips too high (causing your spine to round). Finding the right strength in Incline Plank Pose will help to get your body into a straight line—Mountain Pose—and bring balance to Manipura chakra.

curve is flattened out, the torso caves in, and the fire dies down, leading to introversion and depression.

To balance Manipura chakra, you must find the balance between the rectus abdominis, the erector spinae muscles, and the psoas so that they can work together to hold you up. Then the right amount of light and fire can feed your system and your personal radiance and magnetism can shine through.

ASANAS

Now we will go through a few asanas to illustrate how different movements of the body are affected by the actions of the lower torso. We will apply the principles that you have learned so far in this chapter to a standing pose, forward bend, backward bend, inversion, and twist. Each pose will help you to focus on the alignment of Manipura chakra.

1. TRIANGLE POSE
(Trikonasana)

1. From Mountain Pose, step your left foot back three to four feet, parallel to the back edge of your mat, turning your torso in the same direction. Your right foot should remain parallel to the outside edges of your mat. If you were to draw a line from the heel of your right foot, it would intersect the middle of your left arch. **[A]**

2. Turn your left big toe so that your foot is at an angle of thirty degrees from the back of your mat. Turn your foot in more if your hips are tight, less if they are more open. You should not feel any strain in your knees or hips. Your back foot and knee should follow the direction of your back hip so that they are all facing in the same direction.

3. Check that your ASIS are level and your pelvis is in a neutral position.

4. Inhale and lift your arms out to the side at shoulder height. **[B]**

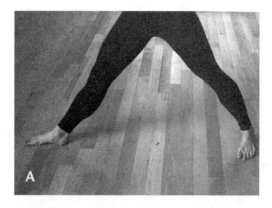

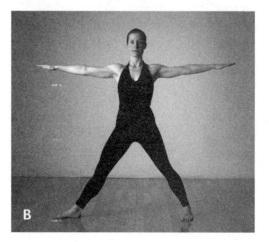

5. Exhale and feel both your feet grounded into the floor. Relax your toes.

6. Inhale, pull your right thighbone into your right hip socket, and externally rotate your right leg. Lengthen your rib cage and extend your right arm out over your right leg as your pelvis shifts toward your left leg. **[C]** You should feel as though your body is moving in two different directions, forward and backward.

7. Exhale. Reach down with your right hand to catch hold of your right ankle, shin, or thigh, or place your hand on a block behind your leg. **[D]** Make sure your right kneecap is drawing up toward your right hip and your knee is straight but not locked; you should feel as if your right shinbone is pressing up into your hand. Go only as far as you can and still maintain the length in your spine and both sides of your body.

8. Lengthen your left arm toward the ceiling, away from your right arm (which is extended down). **[E]** Think of your arms as wings extending out from your spine in a straight line.

9. Bring your left hand to your left hip. Feel how when you firm your right thigh it takes your right hip back, and when you firm your left thigh it lifts your left hip. These actions engage the muscles of the legs and pelvic floor and align the hips so that you can carry your spine in a straight line out over your right leg.

10. Bring your left fingers onto your left shoulder and your left elbow over your left

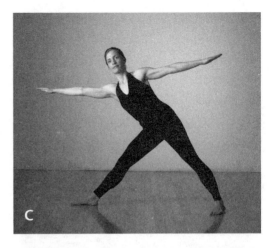

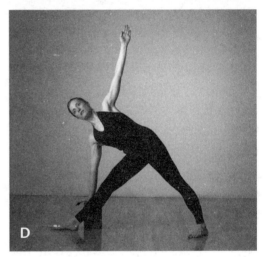

shoulder. Align your left shoulder over your right shoulder and arm. Lift your left hand back up into the air. Feel the space in all of your joints—from the fingers of your right hand up through the fingers of your left hand.

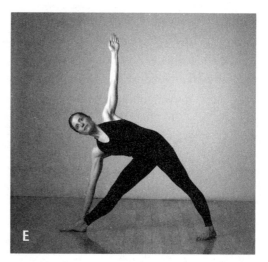

11. Line up your shoulders over your right shinbone and align your hips with your shoulders. Try to bring your whole body into one plane, as if your back were up against a wall. (If you have a tendency to lordosis or to an overly flattened lumbar curve, this will help you to find balance.) If your hips are tight, as most people's are, you may feel a pulling sensation across your pelvis that inhibits you from stacking your hips on top of each other. In that case you can turn your back foot in more and let your left hip drop down slightly, in order to maintain the length through both sides of your torso.

12. Look to a point in front of you, keeping the back of your neck long. If your neck is flexible and it feels comfortable, you can look up to your thumb in the air.

13. Breathe five deep breaths.

14. On an inhalation, use the strength of your leg muscles to lift you back up tall again.

15. Repeat the pose on the other side.

Triangle Pose strengthens your legs and brings a greater awareness of how your legs interact with and stabilize the rest of your body. It shows the importance of positioning your feet correctly in order to find strength and balance in your torso. Always keep your front foot parallel to the outside edges of your mat and your back foot turned in approximately thirty degrees from the back edge of your mat (depending on the openness in your hips). If you draw a line from your front heel, it should intersect the middle of your back arch. With your feet in that position, your foundation has been set. Then you can firm your thighs and concentrate on the correct inward and outward rotations of your legs (your front thigh rotates out, your back thigh in). This will set your hips in the correct position for your spine to lengthen and form the triangle. If your feet and legs are at the wrong angle, this inhibits your ability to lengthen both sides of your body and bring your torso into one plane.

In all standing poses, it is important to get the feet into the right position so that you can balance each leg and activate the pelvic floor. Then you can engage the muscles of your abdomen and back in order to maintain Mountain Pose in your torso and bring stability and balance to Manipura chakra. If your abdominal and back muscles are too weak or too tight, you will tend to arch or round the thoracic spine excessively.

When you are correctly positioned in Triangle Pose, you are using the same principles of leverage that are necessary to hold up a bridge over a river. You can think of the legs and feet as the pillars of support and the torso as the stable structure that allows cars and pedestrians to be carried from one side to the other. When the correct alignment has been set, you can hold up your body firmly and maintain this stability and support in all areas of your life.

2. SEATED FORWARD BEND
(Paschimottanasana)

1. Sit with the spine tall and legs extended forward. Move the fleshy part of your seat back and to the sides to expose your sitting bones, and then balance your sitting bones on the floor as if they were your feet.

2. Bring your legs together and check that your second toe creases, knees, and hip joints are in line. Press with equal strength through all four corners of your feet, keep the inner and outer arches of your feet lifted, and maintain a balance between the inward and outward rotations of your thighs. **[A]** Place your hands on either side of your hips, palms flat on the floor with your middle fingers pointing forward.

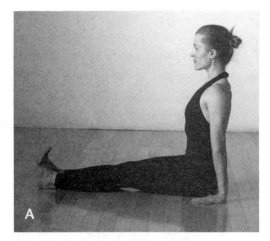

3. Engage your pelvic floor and abdominal muscles, as well as the muscles of your legs.

4. Feel length in your spine and keep your chest lifted as you draw your shoulders away from your ears.

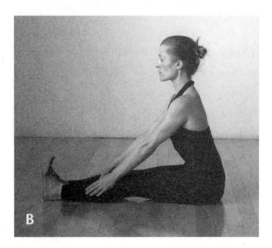

5. Inhale and lengthen your spine, keeping your fingers on the floor. Exhale and extend your hands toward your feet. **[B]** Bend your knees or sit up on a blanket if you feel the upper or lower spine rounding. **[C]** Place your hands on the floor alongside your legs. Or, if you can keep your spine

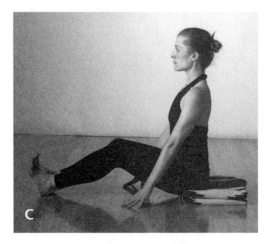

from rounding, place your thumbs and first two fingers around your big toes. **[D]**

6. On each inhalation, feel a lifting in the chest and a lengthening of the spine.

7. On each exhalation, feel your belly draw in and bend forward more deeply.

In Paschimottanasana the legs set up a stable base for the pelvis to initiate the forward bend. It is important to move from the pelvis (rather than rounding your torso), so that you can keep lengthening your spine. You must also engage through the abdominal and back muscles in order to balance Manipura chakra as you continue to extend forward. If the abdominal and back muscles are not engaged, your spine will become overly arched or rounded.

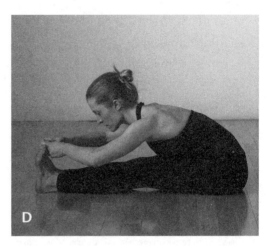

D

3. UPWARD-FACING DOG POSE
(Urdhva Mukha Svanasana)

1. Start by lying on your belly.

2. Place the tops of your feet flat on the floor with your legs parallel and hip-distance apart. Point your toes back and press all ten toenails down into the floor. As in Cobra Pose, rotate your legs inward to create space in your lower back. Place your hands on the floor on either side of your waist. **[A]**

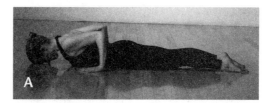

3. Lengthen through your tailbone toward your heels as you engage your pelvic floor and abdominal muscles. Inhale and imagine that your hands are sliding toward your feet as you lift your chest and thighs up off the floor.

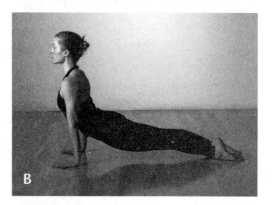

4. Try to straighten your arms (keeping a slight bend in your elbow to prevent locking the joint) and have your wrists, elbows, and shoulders aligned. Draw your shoulders away from your ears. **[B]**

5. Continue to rotate your thighs inward as you bring the back bend into your thoracic spine (feeling your chest open and shoulder blades drawing toward each other). Continue to lift through your abdomen and lengthen your spine and the back of your neck.

6. Breathe five breaths.

7. Slowly lower down.

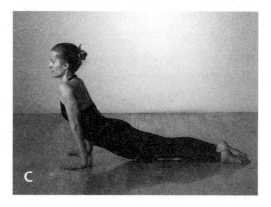

As with all back bends, balancing Manipura chakra in Upward-Facing Dog Pose is critical to protecting the lower back. Most people tend to collapse through the abdomen and compress through the lumbar spine. **[C]**

The abdominal muscles must work with the back muscles to lengthen and gracefully move the back bend into the thoracic spine. If you do not have enough strength to hold the pose comfortably, start in Cobra Pose (the back bend in chapter 3), this time working to feel how the abdominal and erector spinae muscles help to bring the back bend into the thoracic spine.

4. FAN POSE
(Prasarita Padottanasana)

1. Stand with your feet three to four feet apart. The outer edges of your feet should be parallel, which may make you feel slightly pigeon-toed. Your second toe crease, knee, and hip should be in one diagonal line.

2. Feel your weight evenly distributed on all four corners of your feet (base of big toe, base of little toe, inner and outer heel) and your inner and outer arches lifted. Spread your toes wide, engage your quadriceps, and lift through your lower abdomen as you lengthen your spine.

3. Bring your hands onto your hips. Feel as if the sides of your hips could lift up toward your rib cage. **[A]**

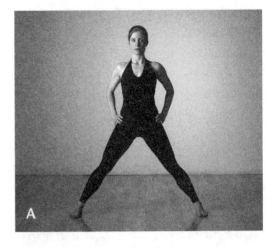

4. With your hands on your hips and your elbows moving back behind you, inhale and lift your chest up, keeping the back of your neck long. **[B]** Engage through your abdomen, your back muscles, and your pelvic floor.

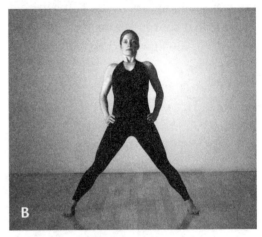

5. Exhale, move your torso forward, and bend down as far as possible. Let the forward bend come from your pelvis rotating forward—do not fold from your rib cage. If your hamstrings are tight, you can bend your knees to help lengthen your spine.

6. Keep your breastbone lengthening away from your hips and keep your chest open; lengthen the back of your neck. Place your hands on the floor with your fingers in line with your toes and your arms bent at right angles. **[C]** If your knees are bent,

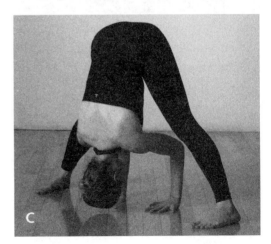

your hands can be slightly in front of your feet. **[D]**

7. Keep lengthening your spine as you breathe five deep, full breaths.

8. To come back up, place your hands on your hips, press firmly into your feet, and bend your knees slightly. Lengthen through your spine as you inhale to come up halfway (so that your back is parallel to the floor). Exhale and lengthen your tailbone down as you draw up to stand. If you feel light-headed, tuck your chin into your chest.

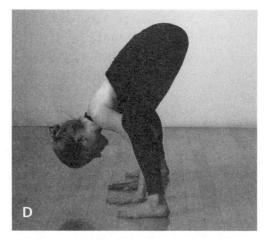

Fan Pose illustrates the importance of balancing Manipura chakra when you are in an inverted posture (with your head lower than your heart). In order for your spine to keep lengthening and your chest to stay open, you must engage both your abdominal and back muscles.

5 . REVOLVED RIGHT ANGLE POSE
(Parivrtta Parsvakonasana)

We twist to the right first to compress the ascending colon, which moves up the right side of the body. We then twist to the left to compress the descending colon, which moves down the left side.

1. Come into a lunge with your left foot forward. Drop your right knee onto the floor (if this is uncomfortable, you can place padding underneath) and bring your hands onto your left thigh. Your front knee should be over your front ankle and your back knee under your back hip.

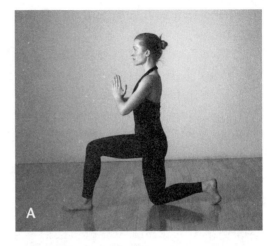

2. Square your hips so that your ASIS are level and pointing forward, and check that your pelvis is not tilting too far forward or backward. Bring your hands into prayer in front of your heart. **[A]** Inhale and lift your rib cage away from your pelvis. Exhale and rotate your spine to bring your right elbow to the outside of your left thigh. **[B]**

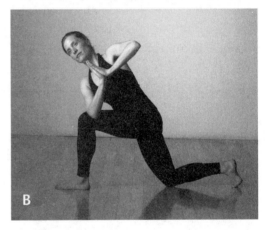

3. Keep lengthening your spine as you rotate around its axis. Draw your left hip crease back and try not to let your right hip drop down in order to keep your hips squared. Let your shoulders draw away from your ears; keep your chest open.

4. If you have your balance, you can lift your back knee off the floor and straighten your back leg. **[C]** Keep your back knee pointing down so that your leg does not rotate open. Find a balance between the inner and outer rotations of both legs. Keep

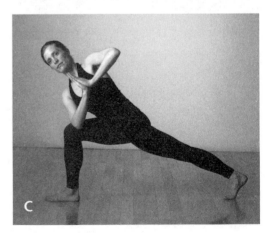

the twist in your thoracic spine, and if you are comfortable, let your head follow gracefully.

5. Breathe five breaths.

6. Bring your hands onto the floor in front of you and switch your legs to repeat the pose on the other side.

Twisting strengthens the muscles around the spine and brings Manipura chakra into balance. When you are in a twist, you are stretching one side and strengthening the other: one side is contracting, and one side is expanding. Twists show that the world is made up of dualities. Seeing both sides balances your fire center and brings clarity to your vision.

FIVE

HARMONIZING EMOTIONS

Anahata, the Air Chakra

ANAHATA, WHICH means "unstruck sound," is the spiritual center of the heart. This chakra is where you begin to tune in to the subtle sound called *nada,* which is the sound of nadi, the pulse of life. From the moment your first cells divide, nadi exists, even before the beat of your heart. Anahata is where you begin to access higher realms of consciousness and experience the finer qualities of sound that exist beyond time and space—what Westerners once called "the music of the spheres."

Anahata chakra is associated with the element of air, which determines what and how you feel. Think of it this way: You start with earth, which is the densest element.

Then water adds fluidity and movement, because earth by itself is stagnant. Add fire and the heat vaporizes the water into clouds, which accumulate in your heart as feelings and emotions. When you hold on to your emotions and get caught up in the senses, the clouds obscure your heart's purity. When you are free of emotional attachment, you can experience a higher consciousness; joy and love can then enter your life.

More than determining your emotions, the air element also dictates your physical perceptions—whether you feel hot or cold, moist or dry. Air also determines the qualities of objects, such as whether they are rough or smooth to the touch. If something feels smooth, there is no air being modulated between your fingertip and the object's surface; an object feels rough if there is a lot of air modulation. Anahata chakra is where you hone your ability to perceive the outside environment: the more balanced your heart, the more refined your perception.

Jiva atman, your personal spirit—your soul, if you like—resides in Anahata chakra. Jiva atman gathers information from life and deals with the material part of you as embodied in the lower three chakras. Anahata chakra is where you begin to move beyond the material self and find a connection to the transcendental self, called *param atman,* which is the inspiration, intelligence, and abundance of universal spirit. Anahata is the portal between jiva atman and param atman: it connects you to the world of the senses, yet gives you access to all the knowledge of the universe! When Anahata is balanced, there is a harmony between external and internal, physical and spiritual; your external life becomes a reflection of your inner values.

Yogananda coined the terms "self-realization" and "God-realization" in relation to atman, or spirit. The beginnings of self-realization take place when Anahata chakra is balanced and you move beyond the qualities of the lower three chakras to connect with jiva atman, the individual part of your spirit. Full self-realization occurs when jiva moves to Ajna chakra and can connect with universal intelligence. God-realization occurs in Sahasrara chakra

(which we will cover in chapter 8) when jiva is liberated (*mukti*) from the world of the senses and moves up to merge with param atman at the crown of the head. Jivan-mukti takes you back to the origins of consciousness to bestow the gift of bliss and oneness with the universe, which in yoga is called samadhi.

Unfortunately, because of spiritual ignorance (avidya) and illusion (maya), our jiva is habitually entangled in our emotions and personal problems relating to the lower three chakras. We suffer because we allow our emotions to govern our lives. We permit our emotional dealings with lovers, friends, and work to define our identity. The limitations of maya and avidya allow us to perceive only a fraction of the truth of existence. We cannot hope to see the whole picture.

When Anahata becomes balanced and jiva can communicate with param atman, spiritual clarity (*viveka*) is restored. When understanding and unconditional love blossom on the inside, you act differently on the outside. Not needing to judge yourself, you cease to judge others.

Unconditional love is not an intellectual process; it is a feeling of fulfillment. It means that you love people regardless of their behavior toward you. You love without looking for recompense. You no longer respond to people according to how agreeable they seem to you. In your relationships you stop trying to be "the lover" or "the beloved" and simply become *loving.* This happens automatically when your heart chakra is balanced and open.

The physical positioning of the heart center can tell you a lot about what is happening to an individual. I have a student whose heart center is so collapsed and sunken that she has become morose and solipsistic. Her need for personal attention and physical proximity is almost unmanageable for others. Her heart has been deflated, she has closed off her emotions, and she has become insensitive to other people's feelings. Married to a domineering man who uses money to control her, she has learned to subordinate her own emotions and desires to her husband's and has forgotten how to listen to her heart. The task I had was to open her heart, both to herself and others.

After she started doing yoga, there was a noticeable change in her. Instead of giving up on her marriage, she is starting to express her needs. This is creating new space for her in the relationship and dramatically changing her life at home. Although she is still a very difficult person and tends to shut down emotionally, I am confident that working with Anahata chakra will help her to live more openly.

On the other hand, when Anahata chakra is overactive, the result is emotional flamboyance. We all know people who address everyone as sweetie or darling regardless of how long they have known them. By putting on a distracting theatrical performance, they can ignore what is going on "backstage" in their lives. Everything becomes a drama. A teacher at my studio was like this. She was always kissing and hugging people, terrified of not being loved—and she always ended up smothering them. As her heart became more balanced, she found clarity and compassion; she saw how she was affecting others and moderated her behavior accordingly. In order to determine whether you have an imbalance in Anahata chakra, consider these questions:

- Do I have trouble finding meaning in my life?
- Is it hard for me to relate to others?
- Am I overly emotional?
- Do I dislike being alone with my feelings and thoughts?
- Am I always looking for others to fill my emotional needs? Do people disappoint me easily?

When Anahata chakra is balanced, you find compassion, which brings kindness and goodwill toward yourself and others. You are able to love without expectations and attachment, from a place of unconditional understanding.

PHYSICAL LOCATION

Anahata chakra is located in the thoracic cavity. It is the energetic center of the heart, which encompasses not only the heart organ but also the rib cage, the sternum, and the front of the spine. To balance Anahata

EXERCISE 1 UPWARD-FACING CAT/ DOWNWARD-FACING CAT POSE (Marjariasana)

1. Kneel on all fours. Place your knees under your hips and the heels of your hands below and in line with the front of your shoulders. The creases of your wrists should be parallel to the front of the mat, and the insides of your elbows should be turned at a forty-five degree angle (in between pointing toward each other and toward the front of the mat).

2. Feel that your spine is lengthening and that your pelvis is in a neutral position. Make sure your fingers are evenly spread, and seek to create space between your neck and shoulders. Squeeze your triceps to externally rotate your upper arm as you ground down through your thumbs and first fingers. **[A]**

3. Inhale and curl your toes under and press them into the floor. Initiating the movement from your pelvis, feel your sitting bones turn up slightly, your thoracic spine arch, and your shoulder blades stabilize on your back as your sternum lengthens forward. Keep your cervical and lumbar curves extended and lengthened, and let your head gently follow the curve of your spine as your gaze lifts slightly. This is Upward-Facing Cat Pose. **[B]**

4. Exhale, point your toes, and feel your shinbones and the tops of your feet pressing more into the floor. Draw your belly in

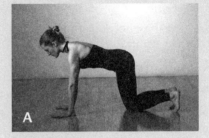

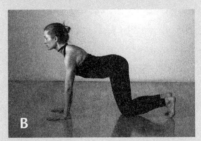

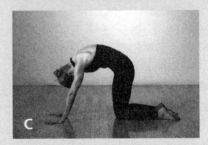

and lengthen your tailbone down toward the floor to create space in your lumbar spine. Feel your lumbar spine rounding and your thoracic curve lengthening, and let your neck and head relax as you gaze toward your navel. This is Downward-Facing Cat Pose. **[C]**

5. Continue to move between Upward-Facing Cat and Downward-Facing

chakra it is important to balance the entire thoracic cavity (front, back, and sides) between your xiphoid process and T12 vertebra (dashed line in figure 12). The muscles that act on the thoracic cavity and work to balance Anahata chakra are the scalenes (neck), pectoralis minor (chest), trapezius (upper back and neck), rhomboids (between the shoulder blades), and erector spinae muscles of the thoracic spine.

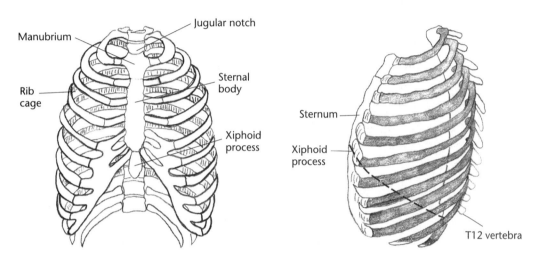

FIG. 11. *Sternum from the front.*   FIG. 12. *Rib cage from the side.*

EXERCISE 1 UPWARD-FACING CAT/
DOWNWARD-FACING CAT POSE *continued*

Cat for five to ten breaths. Try to link your breath to each movement.

In Upward-Facing Cat Pose, it is important to feel your thoracic spine drawing in and the lumbar and cervical spines lengthening (this prevents arching in the lower back). In Downward-Facing Cat Pose, you are rounding the lumbar curve, and the thoracic spine gently lengthens as it follows the expression of that motion. Upward-Facing Cat/Downward-Facing Cat Pose helps you to isolate the curves of your spine and find the movements in your thoracic spine that are needed to balance Anahata chakra.

The thoracic spine is naturally a bit rounded (kyphosis), but when someone is extremely introverted or depressed, the muscles that support Anahata chakra become imbalanced, causing the thoracic kyphosis to become exaggerated, and the thoracic cavity to collapse.

Conversely, if someone is an emotional exhibitionist or excessively sensitive, the thoracic spine becomes overly arched and the chest protrudes, creating the opposite imbalance in Anahata chakra.

Many things we do in life cause us to round the spine as we bend forward: working at the computer, eating, and writing. Even when we relax, we slump, and gravity just makes things worse. Our heart is continually being compressed, which contracts us physically and locks up our emotions. In many older people this turns into hunching. When I was in Scotland a few years ago with my son, I noticed that the traffic signs for old people crossing had pictures of hunchbacked figures with walking sticks. How wonderful it would be if everyone did yoga, and those signs could be replaced with pictures of sprightly, erect septuagenarians!

Any asana can be used to create a balanced Anahata chakra. Back bends make you more energized and extroverted; forward bends are focused inward and calming. In each pose, as in life, you must find the correct balance between the two.

ASANAS

In the following section we will go through five asanas to illustrate how the different movements of the body are affected by the actions of the thoracic cavity. We will feel how to balance Anahata chakra in a standing pose, forward bend, backward bend, inversion, and twist.

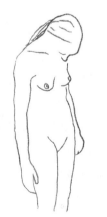

FIG. 13. *Excessive thoracic kyphosis, chest collapsed.*

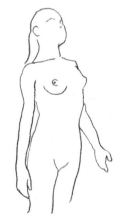

FIG. 14. *Chest too open.*

EXERCISE 2 SPHINX POSE (Ardha Bhujangasana)

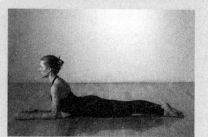

1. Lie flat on your belly.

2. Place your forearms on the floor with your elbows directly under your shoulders. Check that your forearms are parallel and your fingers spread wide, palms down.

3. Bring your legs parallel and balance the inward and outward rotations so that your lower back feels spacious and lengthened.

4. Engage your hamstrings, pelvic floor, and abdomen without squeezing your buttocks together. Rotate your thighs inward, and then lengthen your tailbone. You should not feel any discomfort in your lower back.

5. Feel as though your elbows are drawing back toward your hips (without actually moving them) in order to draw your entire rib cage and breastbone forward and upward. Let your shoulders draw away from your ears, relax your face, and keep the back of your neck long.

6. Place your gaze at a forty-five-degree angle on the floor in front of you.

7. Breathe five deep breaths.

8. Release and lie back on your belly.

Sphinx Pose is ideal for opening and balancing Anahata chakra, because it helps you to isolate the back bend in your thoracic spine. Sphinx Pose strengthens your legs, upper back, arms, and shoulders and counteracts the effects of bad posture. At the same time, it stretches the front of your body and opens up your heart.

1. CRESCENT POSE
(Virabhadrasana II Variation)

1. From Mountain Pose, step your left foot back about four feet and bring it parallel to the back edge of your mat. A line drawn from the heel of your right foot should intersect the middle of your left arch.

2. Make sure your right foot is parallel to the sides of the mat.

3. Bend your right knee so that it is directly over your right ankle. Aim to get your front thigh parallel to the floor. You may need to lengthen your stance to make this possible.

4. Make sure your back leg is straight and your back hip, knee, and ankle are aligned.

5. Position your shoulders directly above your hips so that your torso is perpendicular to the floor.

6. Place your left hand lightly on your left thigh and turn your right palm to face upward.

7. Inhale and lift your right arm and torso up and over your back leg. **[A, B]** Feel both sides of your body and your spine lengthening as you open through your heart. **[C]**

8. Let your gaze turn up toward the hand in the air.

9. Breathe five breaths.

10. Repeat on the other side.

Crescent is a great pose to balance Anahata, because your legs provide grounding for your lower three chakras. From this solid foundation, both sides of your torso can lift and lengthen evenly, and you can gracefully balance your entire thoracic cavity.

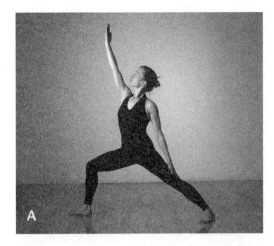

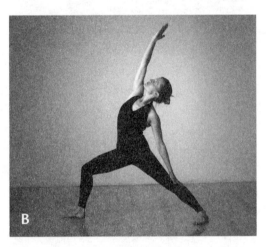

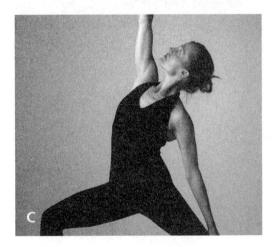

2. HARE POSE
(Hasangasana)

1. Sit back on your heels, then lean forward and place your forehead on the floor, resting your arms by your sides. **[A]**

2. Take your forefingers around the backs of your heels with your thumbs facing down so that you cup your heels in your palms.

3. Lift your seat up in the air and place the crown of your head on the floor as you draw your forehead in toward your knees.

4. Let your abdomen draw in to lift your seat up into the air. Keep your arms straight and feel the stretch around your shoulder girdle and into the back of your neck. **[B]**

5. Be careful not to press and lock your neck. If you have neck problems, do not do this exercise, or modify it by placing your hands on the floor beside your neck to support you.

6. Breathe deeply for five breaths.

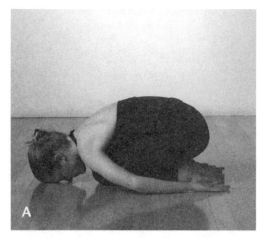

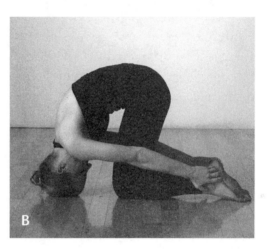

Hare Pose effectively demonstrates how to balance Anahata chakra in a forward bend. In this position the thoracic spine is rounding and you can release tension from the upper back. Whenever I have a client who comes to me with an emotional issue, I know that the upper back and chest will be tight and there will be an imbalance in Anahata chakra. Hare Pose helps to release the tension of the upper back so that you can find space to breathe and open up the back of your body.

3. CAMEL POSE
(Ustrasana)

1. Kneel on the floor with your knees underneath your hips. **[A]** You may want to kneel on a blanket if your knees are sensitive.

2. Bring your hands flat onto the small of your back with your fingers facing upward. If this hurts your wrists, you can turn your fingers to face down. **[B]** Feel your inner thighs squeeze in and back, and lengthen your tailbone.

3. Draw your shoulder blades in and slightly down your back and keep your lower abdomen firm to protect your lower back. Inhale and feel your sternum lifting and opening toward the ceiling. **[C]**

4. Let your head follow the movement without dropping back. (There should be no wrinkles in the back of your neck.) If you are comfortable and your neck is long you can gaze toward the ceiling.

5. On each inhalation, feel that your thoracic cavity expands and your spine lengthens. On each exhalation, deepen into the back bend.

6. Breathe five deep breaths.

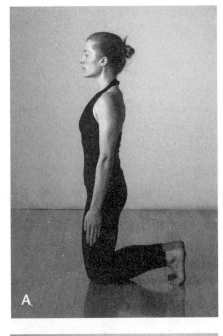

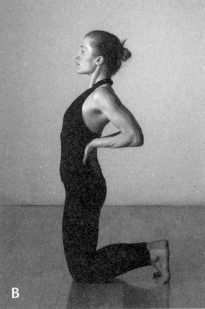

As we have already discussed, the effects of gravity, aging, and emotional tension cause the thoracic spine to round unduly. The more you practice slightly arching through the thoracic curve, the more your heart will open. By balancing Anahata chakra in back bends, you can begin to reprogram your heart!

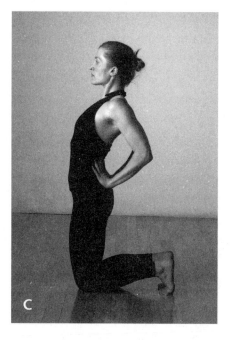

4. FOREARM STAND PREP
(Pincha Mayurasana Prep)

1. Kneel on all fours and then drop your elbows to the floor, directly underneath your shoulders.

2. Bring your forearms parallel, spread your fingers wide, and press your entire forearm, wrist, and hand into the floor. **[A]**

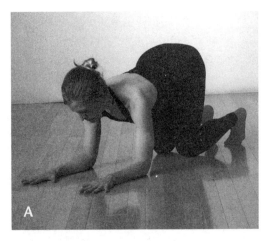

3. Tuck your toes under and begin to lift your knees off the floor, as though you were coming into Downward-Facing Dog Pose. Engage your quadriceps, pelvic floor, and abdomen, and balance the inward and outward rotations of your legs. If you are tight in your shoulders, keep your knees bent and work to open your chest and shoulders. **[B]** Otherwise, begin to straighten your legs.

4. Keep your head off the floor and feel how, as you press into your forearms, you lift your hips even higher into the air. **[C]** Try to keep your chest open and the breath moving freely into both the front and back of your body.

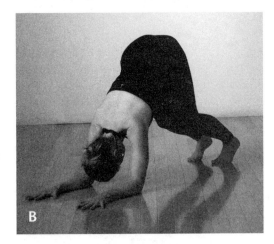

5. Breathe five breaths.

Forearm Stand Prep offers a stable base for the shoulders in order to facilitate the balancing of Anahata chakra. It is very important that you do not excessively arch or round the thoracic spine but find a balance between the two. This will allow your torso to lengthen and your upper chest and shoulders to open in the most elegant and efficient manner.

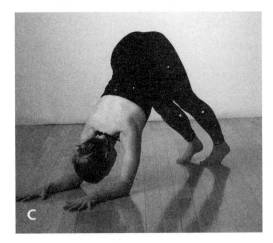

5. REVOLVED HEAD-TO-KNEE POSE
(Parivrtta Janu Sirsasana)

We twist to the right first to compress the ascending colon, which moves up the right side of the body. We then twist to the left to compress the descending colon, which moves down the left side.

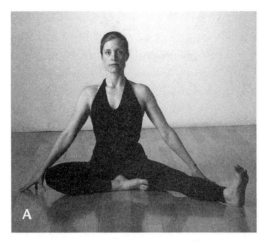

1. Sit on the floor with your left leg extended and the sole of your right foot against your left inner thigh. If you are open in your hips, bring the sole of your right foot in toward your groin. If you are tighter, place your right foot lower on your thigh.

2. Adjust the flesh of your sitting bones so that your weight is evenly balanced (remember, in this pose they act as your feet). Keep your pelvis in a neutral position as you bring your hands out to the sides and rise up onto your fingers. Open across your chest and lengthen your spine as you keep your ASIS squared forward. Let your shoulders relax back and down. **[A]**

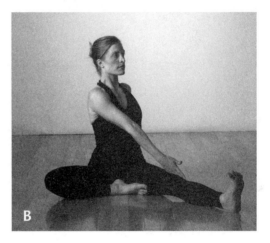

3. Now bring your hands onto the floor in front of you. Engage your abdomen and pelvic floor. Inhale and reach your right arm up into the air. Exhale and slowly twist to the left, placing the back of your right hand against the outside of your left leg or reaching to take hold of the outer edge of your left foot (if you can do this without losing the length in your spine). **[B]**

4. With each inhalation, lengthen your spine; with each exhalation, deepen the twist.

5. Feel your right thigh stable and outwardly rotating as you lengthen forward, maintaining the squareness of your hips.

6. Breathe five breaths.

7. Repeat on the other side.

Parivrtta Janu Sirsasana helps to balance Anahata chakra in a twisting position, because it makes you mindful of lengthening your lumbar spine and bringing the twist more into your thoracic spine. It is important to keep your hips squared and your pelvis in a neutral position to find a balanced opening in your thoracic cavity.

SIX

COMMUNICATING WITH YOUR SPIRIT

Vishuddha, the Space Chakra

VISHUDDHA COMES from the Sanskrit *vi shuddhi. Vi* means "very deep or extreme," and *shuddhi* refers to purification. Vishuddha chakra is the center of extreme purification. When it is in balance, it purifies all of the chakras and brings harmony into your being. Vishuddha facilitates communication between your individual spirit (jiva) and the spirit of the universe (param atman); it connects you to a higher plane of consciousness, so that you can tap into your creativity and intuition and find inspiration in life.

Anahata and Vishuddha chakras are closely related: when Anahata is balanced and open, Vishuddha automatically communicates from a spiritual place and unconditional love shines through. If Anahata chakra is imbalanced, your spirit remains closed and jiva atman operates solely in the world of the senses.

Vishuddha chakra is where we begin to move beyond the attractions of the senses and balance the two energetic forces called the ida and pingala nadis. In Vishuddha chakra ida and pingala come together to move beyond the duality of the material world. When there is union between ida and pingala in Vishuddha chakra, opposites are no longer pulling us apart and we are able to communicate truthfully and with wisdom.

Vishuddha is the headquarters of the element of space. The space element is the backdrop on which all of the other elements are superimposed; Vishuddha chakra underpins your consciousness, your emotions—your very existence. It's an enormously powerful chakra! Vishuddha chakra is analogous to the motherboard inside a computer: it controls the operations of the entire system and permits all of the elements to function in unison. If the motherboard is damaged, nothing will work properly. It is important to keep Vishuddha in balance so that all of the other chakras are optimized.

When Vishuddha is out of balance, you are delayed from reaching your full potential. If it is overactive, your style of communication becomes aggressive, unreceptive, and judgmental; others may feel that you are always "in their face." You are unable to find an authentic voice and are cut off from the inspiration of the universe.

I live in the East Village in New York and park my car in a garage a few blocks from my house. The other day, there was a lady screaming at the parking attendants to hurry up and get her car because she was running late—a perfect example of someone overactive in Vishuddha chakra. With her chin jutting forward, she cut to the front of the line and made a big fuss to the manager, who was backing away from her to create some space between them. After much huffing and puffing on her part, her car arrived, and she got in and drove away,

without any thank you or apology. I'm sure that everyone she came into contact with throughout the day had to suffer the same behavior.

Conversely, when Vishuddha is underactive, you are withdrawn and cannot communicate effectively or enthusiatically. You find it difficult to speak your truth, and because of this your spiritual growth will be hindered.

When I was younger, I was terrified of speaking in front of people. My father was always giving lectures, and I used to say to him, "I don't know how you can sit and talk so much. It just keeps flowing out of you." "One day," he replied, "when Vishuddha chakra is balanced, the same thing will happen to you." He was right. Now, when I need to give a lecture, I just sit down and my communication center starts flowing. I can talk for three to four hours and with total ease. As a kid I thought I would never be able to speak for even half an hour, but with Vishuddha chakra balanced, it feels natural for me to communicate creatively and from a higher place. To determine whether you have an imbalance in Vishuddha chakra, ask yourself the following questions:

- Do others see me as aggressive and overbearing?
- Do I dominate conversations?
- Do I find it hard to speak up for myself?
- Do I live in a way that's true to my core beliefs and values?

- Do I lack inspiration?
- Do I feel connected to my spirituality?

When Vishuddha is balanced, you discover your authentic voice and can be yourself in all situations. Your communication is clear and untainted, and you come to others with compassion and kindness. You have the space to see yourself clearly and can let the divine wisdom of the universe guide each moment of your life.

PHYSICAL LOCATION

Vishuddha chakra is located at the throat. It also encompasses the neck, shoulder girdle, and arms. The muscles that act on Vishuddha chakra are the erector spinae muscles of the neck and upper back, trapezius, rhomboids, muscles of the rotator cuff, pectoralis major, and latissimus dorsi. Balancing all of these muscles is important to bring balance to Vishuddha chakra and enable proper communication.

Interestingly, your ability to communicate is influenced by a little V-shaped bone in your neck called the hyoid bone. The hyoid bone is attached to the thyrohyoid membrane in your throat and serves as the point of convergence for many of the extrinsic muscles of the larynx, in addition to supporting the muscles of the tongue.

The hyoid bone is a signpost for Vishuddha chakra, because it controls how

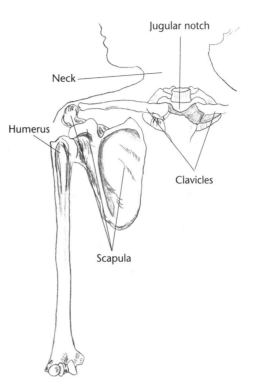

FIG. 15. *Shoulder girdle.*

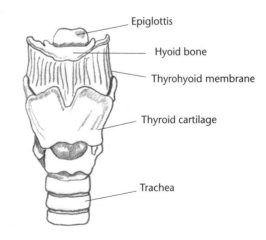

FIG. 16. *Larynx.*

EXERCISE 1 ARM EXTENSION AT THE WALL

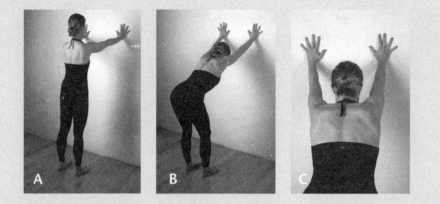

1. Come to stand facing a wall. Place your hands on the wall a little higher than shoulder height and slightly wider than shoulder-distance apart. Spread your fingers wide and check that your middle fingers are pointing upward. [A]

2. Walk your feet back until your arms are straight and your torso is lengthened diagonally away from the wall, while maintaining the natural curves of your spine.

3. Keep your hips, knees, and ankles on top of each other so your legs are straight. If the backs of your legs are tight, you can bend your knees slightly. [B]

4. Press down through your thumb and first finger and feel your forearm bone roll in slightly. At the same time, rotate your upper arm outward to feel your shoulder blades drawing toward each other and slightly down your back. Your shoulders will move away from your ears. [C]

5. Try to find a balance between your forearm bone rolling in and your upper arm bone rolling out. At the same time, feel space between each of your joints and maintain a relaxed neck and shoulders.

6. Let your chest extend toward the floor as you continue to lengthen your spine and maintain tone in your belly.

7. Breathe five breaths.

Arm Extension at the Wall helps you to feel the correct rotation of the arms and positioning of the shoulders and neck. This exercise demonstrates how the position of the shoulder girdle affects the neck and head, and its principles can be used to balance Vishuddha chakra in poses such as Downward-Facing Dog, in which the shoulder girdle acts as the base of support.

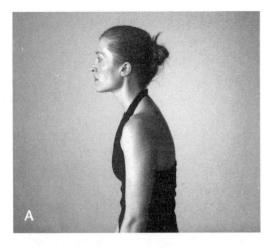

A

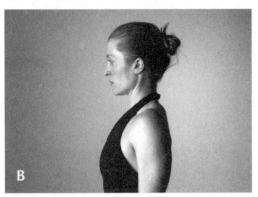

B

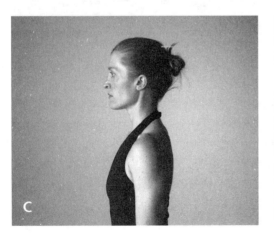

C

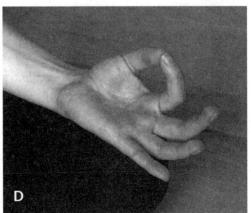

D

your voice is carried. If your hyoid bone juts out because your shoulders have slipped forward, then your communication will be outward, and you will try to control everything in life. **[A]**

If your shoulder girdle is too far back, then your hyoid bone will be drawn too far back, and your communication will be inward and feeble. **[B]**

To balance Vishuddha, it is important to take into account the position of your neck and throat, hyoid bone, shoulder girdle, and arms. **[C]**

Even your hands reflect the balance in Vishuddha chakra by forming yogic hand gestures (mudras) such as jnana mudra when the arms hang freely and your hands are relaxed in seated meditation. **[D]**

When your shoulder girdle and its appendages are balanced, the throat feels spacious. It mirrors an egg shape, with the bottom of the egg positioned at the jugular notch and the top of the egg pointing up to the roof of the mouth. You feel the space element of Vishuddha chakra and your throat starts to feel very broad and open. **[E]**

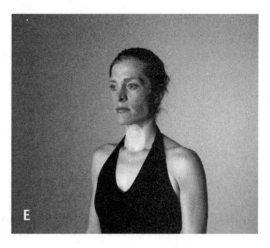

E

ASANAS

Here are a few asanas to illustrate how different movements of the body are affected by the actions of the shoulder girdle and neck. We will apply the alignment of Vishuddha chakra in a standing pose, forward bend, backward bend, inversion, and twist.

EXERCISE 2 VICTORIOUS BREATH POSE (Ujjayi Pranayama)

Ujjayi is a full, complete breath performed by slightly narrowing the vocal cords at the back of the throat. When the vocal cords are contracted, the breath creates a hollow, echoing sound (rather like Darth Vader in *Star Wars*!). Ujjayi makes the breath an audible point of focus, keeps you from breathing too rapidly, and builds heat in the body (due to the friction and increase in effort that this type of breathing produces). Ujjayi also balances Vishuddha chakra by controlling the airflow in the throat and making a sound that purifies the space element.

1. Come into a comfortable cross-legged seat.
2. Place one hand three inches in front of your face with your palm facing you. Place the back of your other hand on your

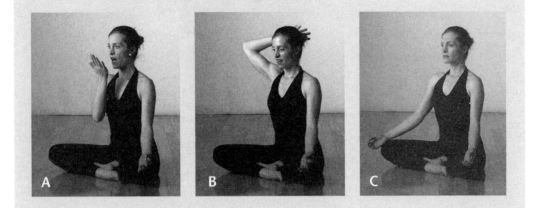

knee with the thumb and forefinger touching, as in jnana mudra. **[A]** Blow air onto your open palm as if you were blowing out a candle on a birthday cake. Feel how the air is cool and dry.

3. Now as you exhale feel the muscles at the back of your throat constrict, and with your mouth open, exhale onto your hand as if it were a mirror you were trying to fog. Feel how the breath is warm and slightly moist. **[A]**

4. Then imagine that you have a mirror behind your head (you can even bring your palm to the back of your head to help you visualize this). As you inhale through an open mouth, imagine fogging the mirror behind you, feeling the same constriction at the back of the throat as you did when you exhaled. **[B]**

5. Once you have successfully created the sound in the throat, it is time to transfer it to the nostrils. So retain the same feeling of fogging the mirror, but close your mouth and breathe in and out through your nose. If you find this challenging, start each inhalation and exhalation with the mouth open, and halfway through the breath, close your mouth. **[C]**

6. Without forcing the breath, pay attention to its sound. Feel the back passage of your throat widening as you breathe in and out. Eventually you will be able to link the breath with movement.

1. UPWARD WORSHIP POSE
(Uttihta Hastasana)

1. Come to stand, feeling all four corners of your feet anchored to the floor. Have your ankles, knees, hips, shoulders, and head stacked on top of each other.

2. Lift your toes, spread them wide, and place them back down. Try not to grip the floor.

3. Reach your arms into the air with your palms facing in. Feel a lifting in the sides of the chest and breastbone. **[A]**

4. Lower your shoulders away from your ears. Feel your collarbones broadening and your spine lengthening. Resist the tendency to draw the shoulders up toward the ears, which is incorrect. **[B]**

5. Feel the sides of the body lengthen all the way up through the outer arm while the inner arm draws down. (This rebalances the shoulder girdle.)

6. Let your head rest gently on top of your shoulders, with the chin neither tilting up nor tucked in toward the throat.

7. Breathe five deep breaths.

8. Lower the arms down to the sides of the body. Feel how the shoulder girdle is stable and your head floats on top.

Upward Worship Pose follows the principles of Mountain Pose with the arms extending up in the air. It helps you to square your shoulder girdle, which is a prerequisite of many standing poses and vital to balancing Vishuddha chakra. As the outside of the arm lifts up and the inside of the arm draws down, you stabilize your shoulder girdle. Once your shoulder girdle is stable, you can lower your arms and feel how your head floats comfortably on top of your spine.

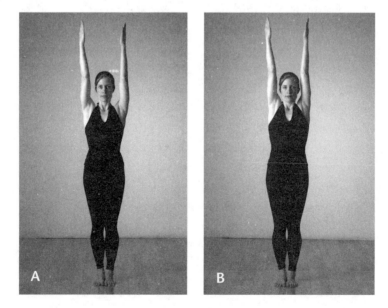

2. PREPARE POSE
(Ardha Uttanasana)

1. Come into a forward bend with your feet together and your belly touching your thighs.

2. Place your hands (or fingertips) on the floor. Engage your quadriceps, your pelvic floor, and your abdomen. Inhale and feel your sternum extend forward, keeping the back of your neck and lumbar spine long and your gaze down and slightly in front of you.

3. Feel your legs pulling backward as you lift your torso parallel to the floor and arch through your thoracic spine. Draw your shoulders toward each other and slightly down your back. **[A]** You can bend your knees and place your hand on your shins or on blocks if your hamstrings are tight. **[B]**

4. If your legs are straight, try to keep your hips over your ankles as you press your heels down into the floor.

5. Keep the back of your neck long as you feel the crown of your head lengthening away from your tailbone.

6. Breathe five breaths.

In Prepare Pose the aim is to extend through the spine so that your torso comes parallel to the floor (in a more flexible practitioner, the thoracic spine will also arch somewhat). Your shoulders are drawn slightly toward each other and down your back so that your chest is open, and the back of your neck is long to keep the throat spacious. There is a tendency to lift the chin too much (creating strain in the back of the neck) or to drop the chin down (constricting the throat). To balance Vishuddha chakra, you want to feel the egg shape resting in the base of your throat and extending up to the roof of your mouth.

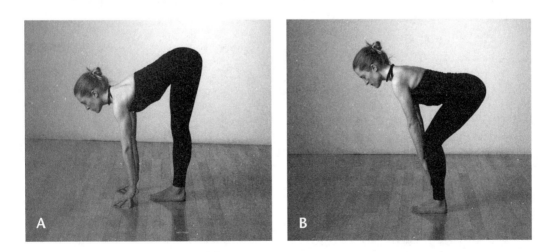

3. FOUR-LEGGED TABLE POSE
(Chatushpada Pitham)

1. Sit on the floor, bend your knees, and walk your feet in until they are about ten inches away from your buttocks.

2. Bring your feet hip-width apart and parallel, and press all four corners of your feet down into the floor. Emphasize pressing into the inside of your foot to feel your inner thighs squeezing toward each other.

3. Place your hands on the floor behind you with your fingers facing toward you. **[A]** If this is uncomfortable, you can let your fingers face away from you. Whichever way you place your hands, make sure that your middle fingers are parallel and your thumb and first fingers are pressing into the floor.

4. Lift the top corners of your chest and draw your shoulder blades toward each other and slightly down your back.

5. Inhale and lift your hips up into the air, firmly pressing down into your hands and feet.

6. Keep your gaze initially toward the tip of your nose and try not to let your seat sag. **[B]**

7. Use the power in your legs to keep yourself lifted, and feel your tailbone drawing toward the backs of your knees.

8. Try to keep your shoulder girdle square and be careful not to jut your chin forward. Maintain a sense of balance in your throat (remember the egg). If it doesn't strain your neck, look up to the ceiling so

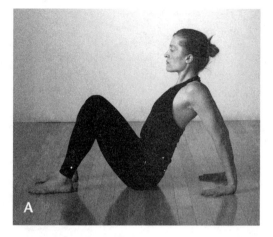

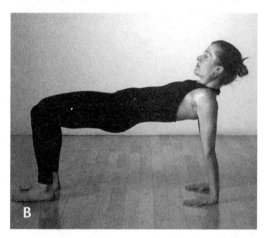

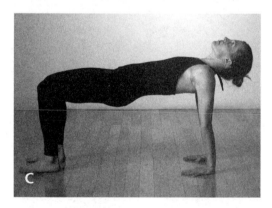

that your hairline and chin are parallel to the floor. **[C]**

9. Breathe five deep breaths. Feel the breath into the sides and top corners of your chest and your belly.

10. If your thighs are level with your abdomen and chest, and the back of your neck is long, your gaze can shift up to your third eye.

11. Slowly lower back down to the floor.

Four-Legged Table is a great pose in which to feel the balance of Vishuddha chakra. Done correctly, it stabilizes the vertebrae in the neck by sustaining the natural cervical curve as you arch the thoracic spine.

4. SHOULDERSTAND PREP
(Salamba Sarvangasana Prep)

1. Lie on your back with your knees bent and feet flat on the floor. **[A]**

2. Press down into your feet to lift your hips up off the floor and slide a block or a thick book underneath you. Lower down so that your sacrum (the triangular bone at the base of your spine) is resting on the block and you have a solid base of support.

3. Feel your shoulder girdle broaden and maintain enough space beneath the back of your neck to slide your hand under. Let your arms extend down so that your hands rest comfortably on either side of your hips.

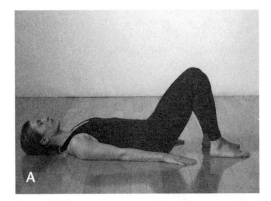

4. Extend your right leg up into the air [B] and then bring your left leg up to meet it. [C] Press up through the balls of your feet as you draw your toes back (it will feel as though you are wearing high heels or driving a car) to activate the muscles of your legs.

5. Breathe five to fifteen deep breaths.

6. Lower one leg at a time, bringing your feet onto the floor.

7. Lift your hips to remove the block and then lower back down.

Keeping your shoulder girdle squared is very important in Shoulderstand Prep (and Shoulderstand), because when the shoulder girdle is square, the natural curve of the cervical spine can be sustained. When the curve of the cervical spine is sustained, the chin and the hairline remain parallel to the floor. The shoulders are away from the ears but not below the level of the shoulder line. If your chin drops down toward your chest or lifts toward the sky, your neck is in hyperextension. You want your body to open around the stable base of the shoulder girdle, keeping space in the neck so that Vishuddha chakra can balance.

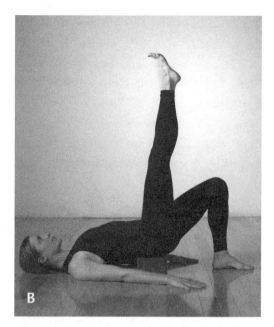

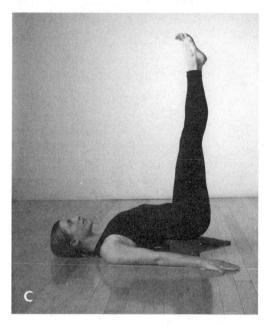

5. SEATED SPINAL TWIST
(Ardha Matsyendrasana)

We twist to the right first to compress the ascending colon, which moves up the right side of the body. We then twist to the left to compress the descending colon, which moves down the left side.

1. Sit up tall on the points of your sitting bones, with your legs straight out in front of you. Balance the inner and outer rotations of your thighs to stabilize your base.

2. Lean forward and feel your sitting bones move back; adjust the flesh around your sitting bones.

3. Come back upright and bring the sole of your right foot onto the floor on the outside of your left knee.

4. Bring your right hand onto the floor behind you (you can stay on your fingertips to help you get length in your spine).

5. Inhale and raise your left arm into the air.

6. Exhale and take your right knee into your left elbow crease as you twist to the right. **[A]** Keep your hips squared as you initiate the twist from your navel. Move the twist up through your thoracic spine and then let your head follow gracefully, keeping the back of your neck long.

7. On each inhalation, feel your spine lengthen and your body expand, creating space. On each exhalation, draw your belly in and move deeper into the space that the inhalation created. If you can maintain the squareness of your hips while twisting, you can bend your left knee and place your left foot in front of your right buttock in order to move into a deeper variation of the pose. **[B]**

8. Breathe five deep breaths.

9. Repeat the pose on the other side.

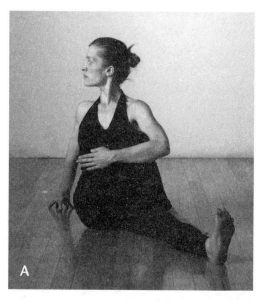

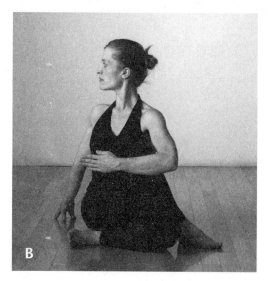

As we have discussed, when twisting it is very important to keep your pelvis stable in order to secure your base. Yet twisting also requires the top of the body to be stable so that the twist can happen in the thoracic spine. Imagine you have a piece of wood in which you are trying to drill a hole. If the wood you are drilling into is not secure at both ends, it will just spin around. In all twisting, the shoulder girdle is square, the neck stays long, and there is space in the throat. When Vishuddha chakra is balanced, the bulk of the twist can happen in your thoracic spine.

SEVEN

ACCESSING YOUR INTUITION

Ajna Chakra, Commander of the Elements

THE WORD *ajna* means "command." Ajna chakra controls the chakras and oversees the management of the elements (earth, water, fire, air, and space). Ajna is like the conductor of an orchestra: it keeps everything running smoothly, so that your chakras can make beautiful music together. If Ajna fails in its task, the chakras will fall out of tune and lose their harmony.

Ajna chakra holds universal intelligence, Mahat, which is the blueprint for creation. Following Mahat's blueprint, Ajna mixes karma with the elements to bring each of your chakras to life.

Karma, derived from the root *kri,* means "action"; it is a mass of energy that is the impetus for your existence and your motivation for growth. Your spirit—atman—chose to take a human birth in order to work out the karma attached to it. Karma determined your rebirth and shapes the experiences of your present and future lives. There are three types of karma:

- *sancita karma* (past karma): the accumulation of karma from past lives that is seeking expression.
- *prarabhda karma* (present karma):

karma that is happening in the present moment. It works off the debts of the past and projects into the future.

- *agami karma* (future karma): karma acquired in the present lifetime that will come to fruition in the future.

These three karmas are always active. How you work through your past and present karma determines whether you release it efficiently or create more karma to deal with in the future. In Tantra, the aim is to move as quickly and smoothly as possible through the karma that life creates, so that you can release it and avoid accumulating more. When karma is released efficiently, it leads to spiritual growth and transcendence; if karma is not released, it continues to recur until it is worked out.

Your ability to move through karma is self-determined. If you are tied to the world of the senses and bound by time on this plane of consciousness, it can take lifetimes to release; if you can go beyond the mind and bounds of time, your karma will release spontaneously.

Releasing karma is similar to releasing a bubble of air from the bottom of a lake. If the bubble moves straight up through the water and pops at the surface, it is released in the most efficient way. If the bubble gets trapped under a rock (the mind and the senses) on its way up, it takes much longer. And if you continue to add more bubbles (of karma) and keep suppressing them, they will never surface.

In addition to governing the distribution of karma, Ajna chakra is associated with manas, the part of your mind that processes the sensory input of the lower five chakras. Through manas, Ajna relates to the world of the senses. Yet Ajna is beyond the duality of the senses; it acts more like an intuitive sixth sense. After originating in the nostrils, ida (left) and pingala (right) nadis move to Ajna prior to their crisscrossing journey through each of the lower chakras, before terminating adjacent to the perineum. As the nadis do not cross in Ajna, it is not thought of as being balanced or imbalanced the way the other chakras are. Rather, Ajna is either open or closed. When the mind is still and all of the lower chakras are in balance, then Ajna chakra opens to communicate with the higher intelligence of Sahasrara chakra and bring you to a place of inspiration, clarity of thought, and healing. When the lower chakras are out of balance, Ajna chakra remains closed and you lose your ability to connect to the divine.

When Ajna chakra opens in meditation, it creates light in your midbrain, like the glowing afterimage you see when a flashbulb goes off. The glow (some people also see patterns and colors) happens when your brain goes into a delta state (the deep sleep rhythm) while you remain awake. Your brain lobes relax, your forehead is smooth, your jaw relaxes, the roof of your mouth lifts, and your eyes gently turn upward, as though you were dozing. In this state you begin to tune in to dimensions of consciousness beyond the mind and can release karma most efficiently.

One day, after three months of practice, I had a profound experience of Ajna opening as I sat in meditation. My mind was still and I experienced samadhi (the state of bliss that is the experience of universal consciousness). I opened my eyes as the sun was coming up, and through the curtain I saw a ray of orange light shining on my father. I closed my eyes and saw the same image of him sitting there. I can still see that image today.

I told him, "I've figured out how film works."

I explained to him the way a shutter works to capture light, and how images are transferred onto film.

My father said, "We're going to go buy you a camera and create a darkroom where you'll be able to do photography. It's just as I told you: when your mind is still, you can know everything."

We went to buy a camera and then set up a darkroom. The first picture I took was of my dad with a beret. I knew intuitively how to develop it, and the picture turned out beautifully. Today it hangs on my nephew Dylan's wall.

PHYSICAL LOCATION

Ajna is located in the midbrain near the pituitary gland. It is sometimes called the third eye, as it is said to be the source of inner vision. Coincidentally, science now tells us that where the yogis located Ajna happens to be the point where the right and left optic nerves cross in the brain, so it literally is a third eye of sorts. Ajna is the meeting point at the space between the eyebrows, the temples, and above the uvula in the back of the throat.

When Vishuddha chakra is in balance and you feel the egg shape in your throat, then the tip of the egg moves up into Ajna and creates a light feeling at the roof of the mouth; your hairline and chin come into balance, and Ajna chakra opens. The relationship between your hairline and chin is vital to creating a proper opening of Ajna, and it requires a balanced relationship between your sternocleidomastoid,

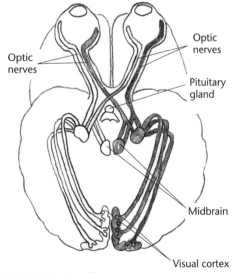

FIG. 17. *Visual pathways.*

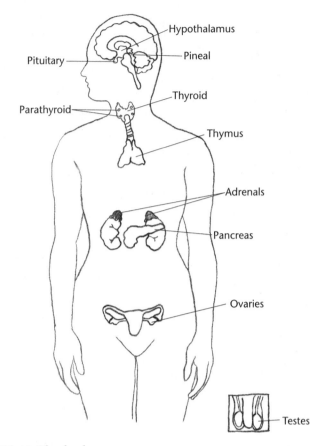

FIG. 18. *The glands.*

your scalenes, and the erector spinae muscles of your cervical spine. If your head is tilted too far upward, Ajna will become too open and you will be spaced out and prone to accidents (although very insightful spiritually). If the head is too far forward (because of stress and tension), Ajna will stay closed. We will explore this opposition in the next exercise (Head Bob).

As already mentioned, Ajna is associated with the pituitary gland. The pituitary is often called the master gland, as it secretes hormones that control the activity of other endocrine glands and regulate various biological processes. Ajna is therefore also thought of as the command center of the glands that relate to each of the chakras. The chakras correspond to various glands as follows:

• Muladhara: the gonads (testes and ovaries), the glands that produce the seeds

EXERCISE 1 HEAD BOB: BALANCING CHIN AND HAIRLINE

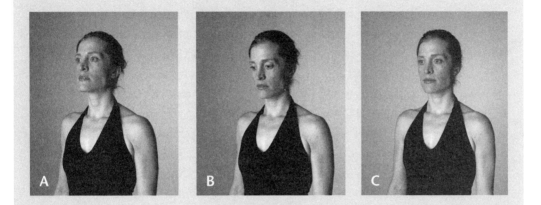

1. Come into Mountain Pose. Let your gaze float upward and your hairline draw backward as you tilt your chin toward the sky. Feel how this creates wrinkles in the back of your neck and inhibits the natural curve of your cervical spine by creating too much of an arch. **[A]**

2. Now let your chin drop down toward your chest and your hairline move down toward the floor. Feel how this compresses your throat and flattens the curve of your cervical spine. **[B]**

3. Find a balance between the two positions so that you maintain the natural curve of your cervical spine, with your head resting comfortably on top of your shoulder girdle. **[C]**

You can open Ajna in any asana when the hairline and the chin are neutral. Finding the balance between chin and hairline will give your head a spacious feeling and allow you to relax your forehead and jaw, making it easier for your consciousness to draw inward and for the inspiration of the universe to flood your being.

from the earth element (sperm and egg) to further life.

- Svadhishthana: the adrenal glands, which sit on top of the kidneys and secrete adrenaline, which governs the ebb and tide of the water in your system (circulation and movement). Adrenaline gives sperm the power to swim to the egg.
- Manipura: the pancreas, located behind the stomach. It produces digestive enzymes and insulin and affects how you metabolize foods and sugars.
- Anahata: the thymus, located in the chest just under the breastbone. It is a prominent factor in the immune system. As we age, the thymus gland naturally shrinks. The older we get and the more stressed we become, the more pressure on the gland and the less strong our immunity.
- Vishuddha: the thyroid, located in the front of the neck, below the larynx. It is like a metronome that regulates the body's metabolic processes. When the thyroid is hyperactive, you become extremely anxious, your metabolism speeds up, and you lose weight. When it is hypoactive, you become lethargic, your tissues swell, and you gain weight.
- Sahasrara: the pineal gland, located at the base of the brain. It controls melatonin, which regulates circadian rhythms.

EXERCISE 2 ALTERNATE NOSTRIL BREATHING (Nadi Shodana Pranayama)

Alternate nostril breathing is a profound technique that creates a balance between the right and left sides of the brain and the sympathetic and parasympathetic nervous systems. The right nostril governs the sympathetic nervous system; it is related to the mathematical, analytical, active, left side of the brain, harnessing Ha, or sun energy. The left nostril governs the parasympathetic nervous system, the creative, free-associative, passive side of the brain, ruled by Tha, or moon energy. Every eighty-eight minutes, one of these nostrils is dominant, then for up to four minutes both nostrils operate equally, and for the next eighty-eight minutes the other nostril becomes more dominant, and so on. You can experience this when your nasal passages are congested: all of a sudden the congestion passes from one nostril to the other.

EXERCISE 2 ALTERNATE NOSTRIL BREATHING
continued

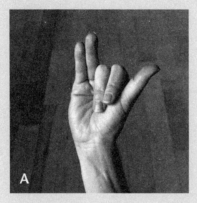

Alternate nostril breathing tricks the brain: it does not know which nostril to make dominant, so it lets the breath flow evenly in and out of both.

On an energetic level, alternate nostril breathing is even more profound. The thumb and ring finger are placed just under the ridge of the hard cartilage in your nose. Staying in contact with the ridge, they regulate the flow of prana into the nostrils. Ida and pingala nadis originate here; as noted earlier, these nadis govern the dualities within us. By keeping the thumb and ring finger in contact with these nadis, you can regulate the flow of prana. When you pause between breaths, you are actually blocking the flow of prana into either nadi and instead are directing the energy into sushumna nadi, the energy channel that runs through the center of the spinal cord. The more you can direct your consciousness into sushumna nadi, the deeper your experience of meditation becomes.

1. Sit in a comfortable cross-legged position. Place the back of your left hand on your left knee with your thumb and index finger forming a circle. This is called jnana mudra, which is an energy seal conducive to relaxation.

2. Take the first two fingers of your right hand to the fleshy part of your palm, letting the thumb and last two fingers remain extended (this is called Vishnu mudra). **[A]** Lift your breastbone to stabilize your

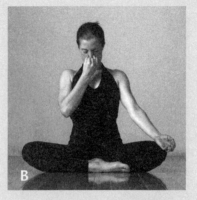

collarbones and shoulder girdle, and let your chin drop down to lengthen through the back of your neck.

3. Lift your right hand to your nostrils and place your thumb on your right nostril and your ring finger on your left nostril, where the hard cartilage and soft cartilage meet. (Note: The thumb and ring finger remain in contact with the nostrils throughout this breathing technique, as they create a subtle pressure that constricts the nasal passage and lengthens the breath.) **[B]**

4. Exhale through both nostrils, block your left nostril completely with your ring finger, and inhale through your right nostril. Block both nostrils and hold your breath as long as is comfortable. When you need to exhale, keep your right nostril closed and let the breath out through your left nostril.

5. Keeping your left nostril open and your right nostril fully blocked, take your next inhalation through your left nostril. Hold your breath in as you block both nostrils, and when you need to exhale, breathe out through your right nostril. This completes one round of alternate nostril breathing.

6. Practice at least six rounds to prepare your mind for meditation, more if your mind is particularly busy. Try to lengthen your breath and, if possible, develop the ability to use the ratio 1:4:2: inhale (1)—hold (4)—exhale (2).

7. When you are finished, lower your right hand back onto your knee, touching the thumb and first finger together. Pause for a few moments and observe the changes in your body.

ASANAS

The following standing pose, forward bend, backward bend, inversion, and twist will help you to open Ajna.

1. TREE POSE
(Vrksasana)

1. Come into Mountain Pose and shift your weight slightly onto your left foot. Spread your toes wide and feel your weight evenly distributed through all four corners of your left foot. Lift your inner and outer arches and engage through your quadriceps as you balance the internal and external rotations of your leg.

2. Engage your pelvic floor and abdomen as you turn your right knee out to the side and draw your right foot up the inside of your left leg. **[A]** Keep your pelvis neutral and your ASIS level, and press your right foot and left thigh against each other with equal pressure. If you have problems balancing, keep the ball of your right foot on the floor or place your foot on your lower leg, against your inner calf. **[B]**

3. Bring your hands into prayer in front of your heart. Feel grounded into the floor as you lengthen up through the crown of your head. Keep the back of your neck long and find the balance between your chin and hairline. Focus your gaze at a fixed point on the wall in front of you to help you balance and quiet your mind.

In Tree Pose, as in all standing poses, you must start with a solid foundation. From there you can work upward to balance each of the chakras. When you have found your balance in Tree Pose and can then direct your focus to opening Ajna chakra, you will feel that your head is floating as the crown lengthens up toward the sky.

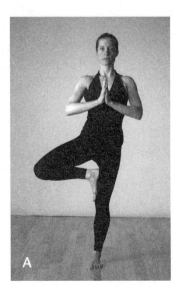
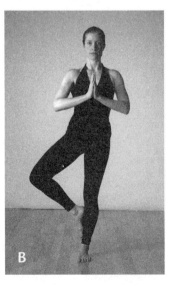

2. THUNDERBOLT SEAL POSE
(Vajra Mudra Asana)

1. Come onto all fours with your hands slightly in front of your shoulders and your knees under your hips. **[A]**

2. With the tops of your feet on the floor, send your seat back to rest on your heels, keeping your arms straight out in front of you. Continue to lengthen your spine as you draw your shoulders away from your ears and feel your forearms lifting away from the floor. **[B]**

3. Rest your forehead on the floor and try to keep the back of your neck long. Find the balance between your chin and hairline. **[C]**

Thunderbolt Seal is a great pose to find the openness of Ajna chakra because it does not require you to focus too much on using muscular strength to hold you up. In Thunderbolt Seal Pose, you can play with the movement of your head in order to bring your chin and hairline into a neutral, balanced position.

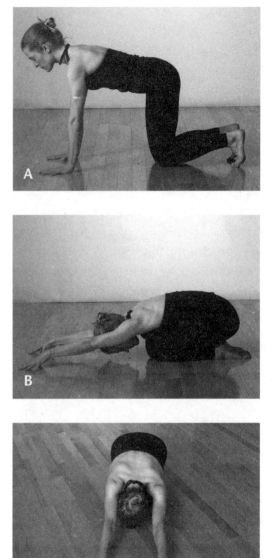

3. BRIDGE POSE
(Setu Bandha Sarvangasana)

1. Lie on your back with your knees bent and your feet flat on the floor under your knees, hip-distance apart.

2. Straighten your arms by your sides and place your hands palms down on either side of your hips. Engage through your abdomen and pelvic floor, lengthen your tailbone, and rotate your thighs inward. **[A]**

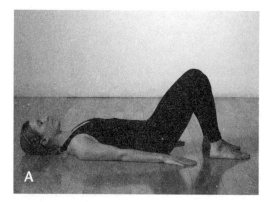

3. On an inhalation, press your feet and hands down into the floor and lift your hips up into the air. If you have neck or shoulder problems, stay in this position; otherwise, lift your chest a little higher and bring your shoulders closer together underneath you, intertwine the fingers of both hands to make a fist, and press your entire arm and fist down onto the floor. **[B]**

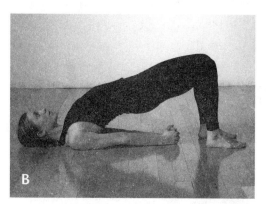

4. Keep pressing down onto all four corners of your feet to engage your hamstrings and lift through your hips. Try not to clench your buttocks.

5. Keep space between your neck and the floor (enough to slide a finger underneath), and balance your chin and hairline.

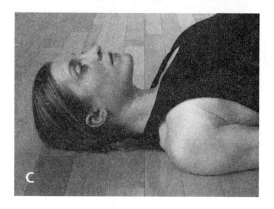

In Bridge Pose, it is vital to balance your chin and hairline in order to protect your cervical spine. If your chin is lifting too far away from your chest, you will compress your cervical spine **[C]**; if your chin is tucked

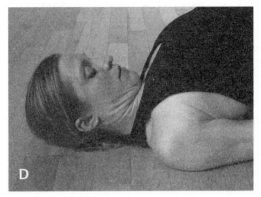

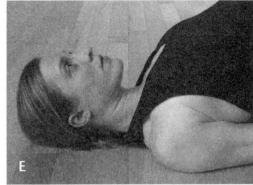

in too much, then the cervical curve will be flattened. [D] Finding the balance between the two will let you focus the back bend in your thoracic spine and allow Ajna chakra to open gracefully. [E]

4. HEADSTAND PREP
(Sirsasana Prep)

1. Kneel on all fours and drop your elbows directly underneath your shoulders.

2. Bring your elbows a little closer than shoulder-width apart.

3. Interlace your fingers and squeeze your palms together. [A] Press your elbows and fist into the floor, and lift your knees up off the floor as if you are going into Downward-Facing Dog Pose. Your head is off the floor and your gaze is at a point in between your legs. [B]

4. Start with your knees bent, and try drawing your shoulder blades in and up your back as you work to create length from your elbows through your armpits to your hips.

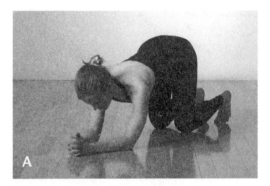

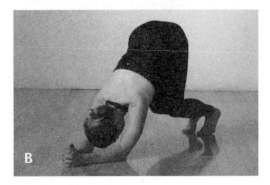

5. Make sure your shoulders are not in front of your elbows and your forearms are pressing your armpits toward your legs. Use your strength to keep your head off the floor.

6. Work your hips higher and higher into the air. **[C]** If you are stronger and more flexible, gradually walk your legs closer to your arms and then work on pressing down again through your elbows and fist to create length in your spine. Try to balance your chin and hairline to create a relaxed and open feeling through your head and neck.

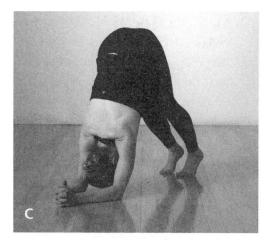

7. Hold the posture comfortably for eight breaths before you walk your legs any closer toward your arms.

8. As you develop strength in this pose, you will be able to breathe comfortably for up to thirty-two breaths. Be careful not to push yourself too far too soon. Keep your breath flowing smoothly and easily.

As in Forearm Stand Prep, you are working here to balance the natural curves of your spine. First find the balance between arching and rounding your thoracic spine and balancing your shoulder girdle, and then carry this up to the crown of your head through the balance of chin and hairline. When you balance your chin and hairline, you can experience the opening in Ajna chakra.

5. RECLINING STRAIGHT LEG TWIST WITH HEAD CENTERED
(Jathara Parivartanasana Variation)

We twist to the right first to compress the ascending colon, which moves up the right side of the body. We then twist to the left to compress the descending colon, which moves down the left side.

1. Lie on your back with your legs together and knees bent, your feet flat on the floor. Extend your arms out to your sides in line with your shoulders.

2. Lift your seat two inches off the floor, shift your hips to the left three to four inches, and place them back down.

3. Keeping your back where it is, draw your knees to your chest and then drop them over to the right—the opposite side to which you shifted your hips a moment ago. This aligns your spine correctly for the twist.

4. Your spine should be in one line from the crown of your head down to your tailbone, and your hips and knees stacked one leg on top of the other. Straighten your legs so that they are extended at a ninety-degree angle to your torso.

5. Check to make sure that your knees stay together. Keep your pelvis and hip structure stable. Extend your right arm to the right and relax your shoulders away from your ears. Do not worry if your right shoulder comes off the floor.

6. Keep your head in a neutral position with your gaze upward. Balance your chin and hairline.

7. Take five deep breaths.

8. Repeat the same sequence on the other side.

As in Maltese Twist, in Reclining Straight Leg Twist you should keep your legs stacked and at a right angle to your spine. In this pose, however, I would like you to focus on isolating the twist in your thoracic spine and keeping your chin and hairline in the neutral position necessary to open Ajna chakra.

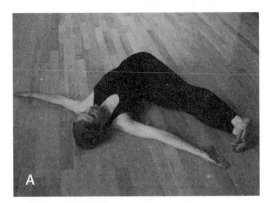

A

EIGHT

RADIATING POWER

Sahasrara Chakra, beyond the Elements

SAHASRARA LITERALLY means "thousandfold," and this chakra is depicted as a thousand-petaled lotus flower in full blossom at the crown of the head. The thousand petals of the lotus relate to the fifty petals found on the lower chakras (Muladhara—four, Svadhishthana—six, Manipura—ten, Anahata—twelve, Vishuddha—sixteen, Ajna—two), multiplied by twenty. Each petal of Sahasrara chakra represents a nadi, through which prana is drawn in from the universe. Sahasrara directs prana into Ajna chakra, where it is combined with karma and the elements and distributed through all of the other chakras to be used in life.

To the ancient yogis, the thousand petals of the lotus signified a number beyond counting: the infinite. Sahasrara is where Shakti first split from Shiva to give birth to consciousness, and it is to Sahasrara that she desires to return. As each of the lower chakras balances and you remove the avidya and karma that keep you trapped in the material world, Shakti gracefully moves up the spine to reunite with Shiva at the crown of the head. With this union in Sahasrara, one can experience samadhi, the bliss of the infinite world beyond life and form.

Sahasrara chakra, like Ajna, is beyond the considerations of the body. It opens when all of the other chakras are in balance, and it remains closed when one is caught up in the illusory world of maya. Sahasrara is located between your hairline and the place yogis call *bindu* (at the back of the crown of the head). When Sahasrara is open, your skull plates feel relaxed and there is a lightness at the top of your head.

Sahasrara is like a screen of consciousness onto which all of the other chakras project—just like the screen at a movie theater. When you watch a film, it is so easy to get caught up in it emotionally. Two hours go by, during which everything you watch seems like reality. Then the movie shuts off, and all that remains is a blank screen. The entire experience was an illusion brought to life by a movie projector and your imagination.

The goal of yoga is to clear Sahasrara's screen so that pure consciousness can reflect clearly and not be obscured by the illusions of maya. The second yoga sutra, *Yogas Citta Vrtti Nirodhah,* explains that yoga happens when consciousness (*citta*) is released (*nirodhah*) from disturbances and movement (*vritti*). When the screen of the mind (citta) is clear of thought and disturbance (vrtti nirodaha), Shiva's inspiration and knowledge floods your being; Shakti is refreshed and replenished and can bring Shiva's wisdom and intelligence (*prajna*) into life.

The first step toward clearing the mind is to practice asanas and bring balance to the physical body. Asanas help to lessen the mind's fluctuations (vritti) and releases karmic patterns (*samskaras*) that have become locked in the body. At the end of each asana practice, it is important to execute one final pose, called Savasana. Savasana is considered one of the most healing asanas, because it allows you to completely integrate your yoga practice and further relax and balance of each segment of your body. As you go through Savasana and focus on relaxing each body part, you stop the electrical impulses to the specific area of your brain (located within the somatosensory cortex) that is associated with that body part, and your mind becomes still.

What yogis have intuitively known for thousands of years is now scientifically illustrated by the figure of a little man called homunculus. Homunculus is a figure that is superimposed on the surface of the brain to show the distribution of the various motor or sensory regions of the body. Each region of the body is represented by the density of touch receptors located there (not by its actual size), so areas that are dense with receptors—such as the fingertips, lips, tongue, and feet—appear proportionately larger than areas with fewer receptors, such as the torso or legs. The little man has big feet and hands, huge lips and tongue, and a small torso and legs.

The yogis have taught Savasana as a way of relaxing each body part, with particular attention paid to the areas that are dense with receptors. Once relaxation is achieved, the brain ceases all superfluous activity and you can experience complete surrender.

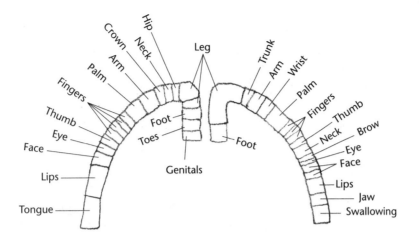

FIG. 19A. *Sensory receptors in the brain.*

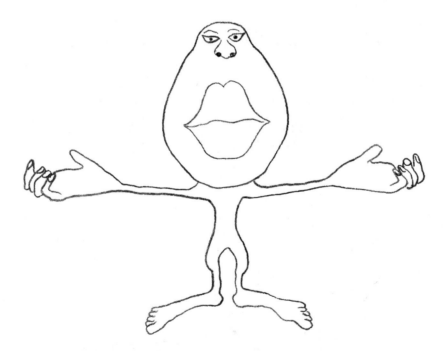

FIG. 19B. *Homunculus.*

CORPSE POSE
(Savasana)

1. Lie down on your back with your knees bent and your feet flat on the floor. Draw your tailbone down toward your heels to find length in your lower back. If you have a sensitive lower back or too much pelvic tilt, you can slide a bolster underneath your knees. Otherwise, extend your legs down along the floor. You may want to cover up with a blanket and/or use an eye pad to deepen your experience. Let go of the echoey-sounding ujjayi breath and breathe freely.

2. Imagine that you have a line drawn down the center of your body and that the right and left halves of your body are evenly distributed on either side of it. With your knees about a foot apart, allow your feet to drop open to the sides. Notice the alignment of your ASIS, sitting bones, pubic bone, and tailbone, and adjust yourself so that your hip bones are level and your

pelvis is in a neutral position. Balance your rib cage so that your thoracic spine can settle into the floor. Draw your shoulder blades toward each other and down so that your shoulders are away from your ears and the edges of your shoulders slope down toward the floor. Place your hands, palms facing up, about six to eight inches away from your hips so that your arms extend out in a V. Let your fingers be slightly curled so that they are not touching one another. Rest the back of your head on the floor or place it on a blanket if that is more comfortable. Balance your chin and hairline. Close your eyes, feel your eyelids meeting and resting gently. Now we will scan through the various segments of your body to systematically release any residual tension.

3. Bring your awareness to your feet. Relax your right big toe, second toe, third toe, fourth toe, and little toe. Repeat on your left toes. Relax your right foot and then your left foot. Relax your right leg and left leg.

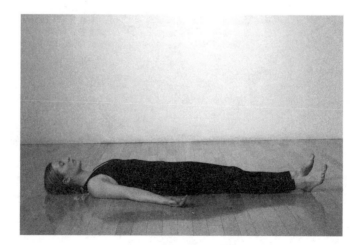

4. Relax your pelvis and genitals.

5. Relax all of the muscles of your abdomen and lower back.

6. Relax your upper torso.

7. Relax your entire right palm, and then your right thumb, index finger, middle finger, ring finger, and little finger. Repeat on the left hand.

8. Relax your right forearm, elbow, and upper arm, and then your left.

9. Relax your shoulder girdle and neck.

10. Relax your eyes and let your eyeballs sink deeply into their sockets. Relax your nose.

11. Relax the rest of your face and your jaw. Relax your lips, allowing them to separate slightly.

12. Relax your tongue and feel the roof of your mouth soft and lifted.

13. Stay in Savasana for ten to fifteen minutes. Try to continue in a state of deep relaxation.

14. To come out of Savasana, roll over onto your right side and spend ten to twenty breaths in the fetal position before slowly sitting back up. Use the support of your arms to raise your body, without tensing your neck and back. Let your head come up last.

In Savasana, your body goes into a state called *yoga nidra* (sleepless sleep), which allows any residual tension you may be holding to drain away so that your body can heal itself on a profound level. As your breath goes quiet and your body becomes still, your attention systematically moves away from the world of the senses and your mind moves into a state of relaxed awareness. Gradually, your brain waves slow down. First, your brain goes from beta waves (waking state) to alpha waves. Alpha waves are the waves you experience when you are falling asleep or taking a "power nap." Scientists call this state hypnagogic, when physical, mental, and emotional relaxation occurs. The hypnagogic state usually lasts from a few seconds to a few minutes. In yoga nidra, the goal is to suspend the alpha state as you stay awake, and then move into the even slower theta waves. Theta waves are the waves of dream sleep, when the unconscious mind begins to release its memories, suppressions, and karmic patterns (samskaras). This state can be very healing if you can release what is in your unconscious without getting attached to what is coming up or trying to interpret it. When all of your samskaras have been released, your brain goes into delta waves, which are the waves experienced in deep sleep. It is when you are awake in deep sleep that you experience samadhi. For most of us, it is hard to get into delta rhythms in Savasana, because we fall asleep. A seated meditation position is preferable, because it keeps your body slightly active while your brain waves decrease in frequency.

AKASHAS

I will lead you through a comprehensive chakra-balancing seated meditation on the online audio recording, but first I want to explain a little about what happens when your consciousness draws inward during the meditative state. The yogis describe in detail various spaces, called *akashas*, that consciousness returns to when it migrates from the lower chakras (the finite world of the senses) to Ajna and Sahasrara (the infinite world of universal intelligence).

- *Cit akasha.* From the world of the senses of the lower chakras, the first space the consciousness gravitates to is Ajna chakra, at the midbrain.
- *Dahar akasha.* When consciousness is complete in Cit akasha, it moves to the space between the lobes of the brain and a transformation process occurs (emotions surface and the true self emerges—beyond the illusions of maya and the vritti of the mind—sometimes accompanied by a physical reaction). In this space you must surrender and practice *bhakti* (devotion) to allow the brain lobes to feel relaxed.
- *Param akasha.* When the brain lobes feel relaxed, consciousness moves to the space between the brain and the top of the head. Here mind and thought have been transcended, and you experience Param (the Supreme). In Param akasha,

Sahasrara chakra opens and the pineal gland secretes serotonin (a mood enhancer), which gives the feeling of going beyond the physical.

- *Atman akasha.* After you reach Param akasha, consciousness then moves to the top of the head, called Brahma Randa (located at the fontanel). Brahma Randa is your connection to the universe; in Atman akasha it softens, opens, and expands outward to connect to the intelligence of Maha akasha.
- *Maha akasha.* The realm of Universal Intelligence. Your consciousness moves completely beyond the physical to radiate outward like an auric field.

It is very important to put aside time every day to sit and allow Sahasrara chakra to open and connect with Atman and Maha akashas. Then you can let samskaras surface and release them in the most productive, profound, and graceful manner. When Sahasrara opens and the wisdom of Maha akasha is available, you experience samadhi. Once you have reached samadhi and can bring the oneness of your experience and its inspiration, intuition, and healing back to be used in this life, it is called *Samyama*, which means "bringing the wisdom of the universe into life." Samyama brings about the possibility of *siddhi*s, or miracles.

The *Yoga Sutras* make mention of siddhis such as levitation, the ability to produce another body, and telepathy. Other, more commonplace siddhis include heightened intuition and what we call the sixth sense. In order to be able to deepen your meditative experience and reach samadhi to bring it into life through Samyama, you must be able to sit comfortably for at least eighteen minutes. At first this may seem difficult, but if you are comfortable, patient, and practice meditation regularly, eighteen minutes will eventually seem to pass in an instant. The following instructions will help you to find a comfortable seat to prepare for meditation.

SEATED MEDITATION

1. Come into a comfortable cross-legged seat with one ankle in front of the other (we call this pose Sukhasana, "easy seat"). If you are new to meditation, you may want to sit with your back against a wall to help keep your spine long.

2. Check that your knees are not raised higher than your hips. You can sit on a blanket or a yoga wedge if your hips are tight, in order to let your knees drop down.

3. Draw the fleshy part of your buttocks back so that you can balance your weight evenly on your sitting bones.

4. Find your pelvis in a neutral position (not tilting too far forward or too far back) with your ASIS pointing forward. Feel a slight drawing-up of your pelvic floor.

5. Lengthen from the base of your spine up through the crown of your head. Try to maintain the natural curves of your spine.

6. Turn your palms to face up and bring the thumb and first finger of each hand to touch. Let your arms relax.

7. Relax your shoulders and feel your head floating comfortably on top of your shoulder girdle. Soften your face and jaw.

Once you have found a comfortable seat, you are ready for meditation. The following chapter will explain the various components of the chakra-balancing meditation that you will find on the audio recording on Shambhala's website.

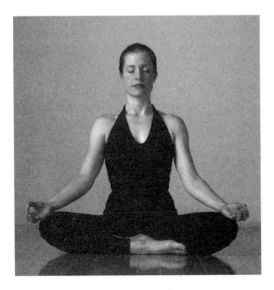

NINE

MANTRA AND YANTRA

IF YOU ARE new to yoga, and even if you have been practicing for a long time, you may find the practice challenging in numerous ways, physically and psychologically. Not only are your muscles learning to speak in different ways, but many of the concepts you are exposed to originate in an entirely different culture. For some people this can be overwhelming! Many yoga practitioners, myself included, translate Sanskrit concepts into English to make them more accessible. But Sanskrit sounds, and the ideas behind those words, are still vital components of yogic teachings. Let me explain why.

Sanskrit evolved as a language with a purely spiritual purpose. Its primary aim was to explain the process of yoga, which, as I mentioned earlier, can be literally trans-

lated as "to yoke." The word *yoga* is also used to describe the experience of yoga, the blissful state of oneness with universal intelligence called samadhi.

Like *yoga,* each term in Sanskrit has such a profound meaning that it is very difficult to find its equivalent in English. Translating a word from Sanskrit is like opening a folder in your computer: inside there are more folders containing more information. In using a single Sanskrit word, I am describing a world. Terms such as *yoga* and *chakra* are complex and profound, and the greater your understanding of them, the deeper your practice will be.

I was first exposed to the practice and language of yoga as a child; if you are encountering it for the first time as an adult, it may seem strange and new. I was recently in a shop in New York whose Indian owner had set up an altar in the back to the goddess Durga, sitting on a tiger, and Ganesha, the elephant god—all surrounded by burning candles! I smiled to myself, wondering how such peculiar deities must look to a Westerner. Don't think that the owners were actually worshipping a woman on a tiger and an elephant man! The altar was there as the receptacle of their prayers. Each deity represents certain qualities and characteristics. Durga, with her spears, represents the ability to slice through the jungle of life; Ganesha symbolizes the removal of life's obstacles. These deities represent a consciousness alien to the West: they celebrate the elements both within us and surrounding us. No wonder people often have trouble understanding the philosophy of yoga at first.

Yoga originated thousands of years ago when *rishi*s, or ancient seers, trekked high up into the Himalayas to find truth; their Hindu deities were worshipped as personifications of transcendental reality. Under the influence of the altitude, breathing techniques, and prolonged meditation, they would go into trances; certain drugs were also employed to liberate them from normal perception. In their altered state they would start chanting sounds and seeing shapes. Over the years the rishis attracted followers who came to live in the mountains with them. Gradually, their experiences and understanding of the "other side" of conscious-

ness were compiled and set down. Today there are different explanations of certain concepts (such as the chakras) because each rishi handed down a unique interpretation, but the wisdom underlying it all originated from and takes us back to the same place.

The rishis used nature to explain their experience. Yoga is filled with images of animals and flowers, shapes and colors from the natural world. They are symbols of the energy inherent in natural forces, and we can use them to tune in to different qualities of energy in our life. Each chakra has a shape (yantra) and a sound (mantra); these are used, just like asana practice, to balance the elements and access the same subtle dimensions of yoga that the rishis experienced thousands of years ago.

I will lead you through a comprehensive chakra meditation on the online audio recording, but first I would like to explain a little about the different mantras and yantras that we will be using. If all this seems strange at first, I urge you to keep practicing and have faith. I assure you that these sounds and shapes, if used consistently, will bring you the balance that you seek.

THE POWER OF MANTRA

Mantra comes from the root words *manas,* "mind," and *tra,* "tool." In Tantra, mantras are used for psychological, physical, chemical, emotional, and spiritual stability and transformation: they work in the realms of consciousness beyond our senses and are used to expand the mind and free it of obstacles. It is only when you expose yourself to the power of vibrating sounds that you can comprehend their profound effects. Everyone has experienced the different emotional responses brought on by music that is soothing—and the opposite! Flute or sitar music brings your energy up to the crown; heavy rock draws you down to the base. Different sounds have different effects.

The repetition of the vibrations of various mantras can help you to tune in to the different frequencies of energy in the universe, in order to effect and transform energy on this plane of consciousness. Each chakra has a specific base sound, or Bija mantra, that can be used to balance it. When you look at a visual representation of a chakra, you can see the Bija mantra represented as a Sanskrit letter at the center of it. The Bija mantras are:

Muladhara: LAM
Svadhishthana: VAM
Manipura: RAM
Anahata: YAM
Vishuddha: HAM
Ajna: KE-SHAM
Sahasrara: OM

When I was younger and the swamis were teaching at my house in South Africa, I asked them why these particular sounds were used. They sat me down and gave me the following exercise:

1. Draw your awareness to Muladhara chakra at your perineum. Make the sound *luh* a few times and feel how Muladhara chakra jumps. To stretch and activate the sound, add *am*. Resonating the mantra LAM LAM LAM balances Muladhara chakra.

2. Now bring your awareness to Svadhishthana in the bowl of your pelvis. Articulate the sound *vuh* a few times. Feel the vibration in your pubic area and sacrum. Add *am* to lengthen the sound. VAM VAM VAM is the mantra used to balance Svadhishthana chakra.

3. Take your awareness to your navel. Say *ruh* a few times and feel the vibration there. Chant RAM RAM RAM to balance Manipura chakra.

4. At your heart center, feel the vibration when you make the sound *yuh*. You can even place your hand on your chest and feel it vibrate. Chant YAM YAM YAM to balance Anahata chakra.

5. Move up to your throat and say *huh* a few times. Place your hand on your throat to really feel it. HAM HAM HAM will balance Vishuddha chakra.

6. For Ajna say *ke-shuh* a few times. Feel the energy moving up from your throat (on *e*) to the middle of your brain (on *shuh*). Chant KE-SHAM KE-SHAM KE-SHAM to bring your consciousness from Vishuddha up to your midbrain to open Ajna chakra.

7. Move the awareness to Sahasrara at the crown and chant OM OM OM.

I will lead you through this technique in the comprehensive chakra-balancing meditation on the online audio recording. You can also use the Bija mantras to help work through any problem that you have in life.

For example, in Muladhara you can look at the problem in terms of what it has to do with earthen qualities—stability, strength, and so on. What are its roots? Then use LAM to release it.

In Svadhishthana, you can deal with the water element. How are you circulating the problem in your life? How is it distributed? What is its movement? Use VAM to release it.

In Manipura, add heat to transform the problem using the mantra RAM.

In Anahata, you can bring up all of the feelings associated the problem and release them with the mantra YAM.

Vishuddha distances you from the problem so that you can see it clearly and send it back to the universe with the mantra HAM.

Ajna and Sahasrara allow the problem to release out of you using KE-SHAM and OM.

THE POWER OF YANTRA

When Shiva and Shakti move away from each other to create form, pure white light is drawn in from Sahasrara and then mixed with each element to create the background color of each chakra. The pure white light in Sahasrara transforms into violet in the third eye, and then down through the colors of the rainbow: blue in Vishuddha, green in Anahata, yellow in Manipura, orange in Svadhishthana, red in Muladhara. These colors are the background and base to each chakra, each one corresponding to a chakra's elemental qualities. Visualizing the background color relevant to each chakra will assist in balancing it (red balances earth, orange balances water, and so on).

In addition, each chakra has a shape, called a yantra, that when visualized can bring balance and harmony to each of the elements. The yantras of the chakras stabilize each element and bring them to their perfect vibratory frequency. Yantras are tools to help you to withdraw your consciousness from the outer world and go beyond the normal framework of the mind into altered states of consciousness and ultimate liberation.

Traditionally, each chakra is seen in the form of a lotus made up of a certain number of petals, with the yantra at its center.

Muladhara

The yantra to balance Muladhara chakra is a golden square. Gold is very solid and pure; it represents the precious metals of the earth. The square is a shape of stability. The four sides of the square represent the earth and its four directions: north, east, south, and west. The animal in Muladhara is an elephant with seven trunks pointing in every direction. The trunks represent the seven *dhatus*, or structural elements of the body as defined in ayurveda: (1) *rasa* (plasma), (2) *rakta* (blood), (3) *mamsa* (muscle), (4) *meda* (fat), (5) *asthi* (bone), (6) *majja* (bone marrow and nerves), and (7) *shukra* (reproductive tissues that produce *ojas*, the vital nectar that is the essence of all the other dhatus). They also represent the senses out of control. Muladhara chakra has four petals.

Svadishthana

The yantra to balance Svadhishthana chakra is a silver crescent moon with its tips touching. The moon governs the water element and the tides. The inner circle has petals that represent the unconscious forces buried deep within. The outer circle has petals that symbolize the outward expression of the conscious mind.

The animal that appears in Svadhishthana is a crocodile, which represents the nature of sexual energy. A crocodile can lie dormant and placid in the water, yet if it is disturbed, its mouth will snap open to attack. The same thing happens with sexual energy: it will be quiescent and then suddenly become aroused. Svadhishthana chakra has six petals.

Manipura

The yantra to balance Manipura is a red triangle pointing downward. The color red represents fire and heat. The triangle is the radiance of the fire energy and metabolism located in your navel. Manipura chakra's animal is a ram. When the heat in your system is balanced, you have energy and proper perspective of the ego (like a ram placidly grazing). If you have too much heat, you become like a ram that butts when challenged. When you have too little heat, you are like a ram that has lost his horns and is rendered powerless. Manipura has ten petals.

Anahata

Anahata's balancing yantra is two powder blue overlapping triangles, one pointing up, one pointing down. This shows where jiva atman resides and how jiva is the consciousness that can deal either with the material self (triangle pointing down to the lower three chakras) or the transcendental wisdom of param atman (triangle pointing up to the higher chakras). Powder blue is the color of air and the sky, which symbolizes the expansiveness needed for the heart to open. The animal in Anahata is a deer with luminous, soft eyes that represent the concept of unconditional love. Anahata chakra has twelve petals.

Vishuddha

The yantra to balance Vishuddha chakra is a white circle with a smoky gray oval shape (like an egg) inside it. The top of the oval is in the roof of the mouth and the bottom is in the jugular notch. This yantra takes the energy from your throat through to Ajna.

The animal for Vishuddha chakra is an elephant whose trunk points upward to show mastery of the senses. Vishuddha has sixteen petals.

Ajna

Ajna contains five beams of white light that come from Sahasrara. It is also sometimes depicted as a violet-colored eye. The third eye transcends all animal attributes. Ajna has two petals that command ida and pingala nadis and represent the duality of the world of the senses.

Sahasrara

Sahasrara's yantra is a thousand-petaled lotus. If you take the fifty nadis (represented by petals) that are on the lower chakras, each one of them multiplies twenty times and connects to the thousand petals of the crown. Sahasrara chakra transcends every aspect of life and physical form.

TEN

A FINAL WORD OF ENCOURAGEMENT

THERE IS AN EXCELLENT reason to take up yoga: it helps you become the person you want to be. In this, I believe, the physical and spiritual practice of yoga is unique. That is why I have been doing it for more than forty years. It is the only way I have found to put aside the constant pressures of daily life and return to a state of balance, an equilibrium of body and mind that belongs to everyone but is often lost when we are trapped in the world of the senses. There is joy and peace to be had in this life. It can be discovered through the art of yoga.

Nobody who is overweight, stressed out, or addicted feels the way he or she truly wants to feel. I should know—I have suffered from all of these difficulties. I did not cure myself in a day, and neither will you. But if you continue to practice, the practice will eventually become a part of you.

If you are new to physical exercise, have been inactive, or have a preexisting medical condition, please check with your doctor before you start this or any other exercise program. Go slowly at the beginning. Don't rush your progress—the results will soon surprise you.

Practice every day if you can. Sometimes the hardest part of the practice is getting to the mat, but it is much more beneficial to practice for fifteen or twenty minutes every day than an hour and a half once a week. Connecting with yourself every day leads to rejuvenation and healing.

I like to practice first thing in the morning, before the day becomes too demanding. I find morning yoga really improves the quality of my day. But if you prefer to do it at midnight, do it then, by all means! Just as long as you do.

The chakra system is a very powerful yogic tool that offers a way to explore and modify the self. Gaining an understanding of the energy centers and their five elements will help to promote the beneficial changes that you seek in your life.

If you can spare the time, the daily asana sequence outlined in the appendix is a well-rounded routine that you can use to create strength and flexibility. It will open you up to sit comfortably for the chakra meditation on the online audio recording.

For a shorter practice, choose one of the sequences designed to target a specific chakra that needs your attention and then practice a meditation using that chakra's mantra and yantra. For example, if you are undergoing emotional upheaval, the sequence designed to target Anahata chakra will help return you to stability.

If you only have a few minutes to practice, choose one or two poses according to your immediate needs. If you need to feel grounded, practice Mountain Pose to bal-ance Muladhara chakra. Feel your feet connecting to the earth and then work to stabilize each segment of your body. (You can do this while waiting in line at the bank or taking the elevator up to your office.) If you need to communicate more effectively, practice one of the poses recommended for balancing Vishuddha chakra. (Arm Extension at the Wall is convenient to do in many situations.) If your physical movement is restricted, merely closing your eyes and feeling the smoky gray egg shape at your throat, while silently vibrating the mantra HAM, will pay dividends.

If you are unable to complete any kind of physical practice, you can use the chakra meditation on the audio recording to balance each energy center, or use individual mantras and yantras to work with the more subtle energetic aspects of a specific chakra—anywhere, anytime.

Yoga is not a competitive sport. There is no race, no time limit, no struggle. Practice with intent, but let the results happen naturally. Be kind to yourself and enjoy each precious moment.

With warm best wishes for your journey.

Namaste

APPENDIX
Putting It All Together

The following sequences form a daily routine that can be used to balance all of the chakras. Keeping in mind the principles explained throughout the book, feel how each asana can help you to balance all of the chakras.

Each asana should be held for the duration of five complete breaths unless otherwise indicated. For asanas that are done on right and left sides, hold the pose for five breaths on each side.

FULL ASANA DAILY SEQUENCE

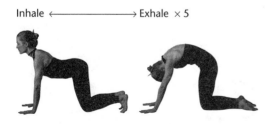

Inhale ⟵⟶ Exhale × 5

Inhale ⟵⟶ Exhale × 5

1. Upward-Facing Cat/Downward-Facing Cat Pose (Marjariasana)

2. Upward-Facing Cat Pose (Marjariasana)/ Thunderbolt Seal Pose (Vajra Mudra Asana)

FULL ASANA DAILY SEQUENCE CONTINUED

Inhale

Exhale and stay for 5 breaths

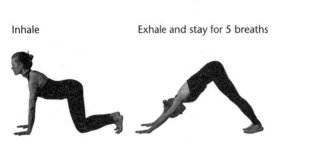

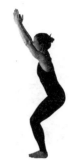

3. Upward-Facing Cat Pose (Marjariasana)/
Downward-Facing Dog Pose (Adho Mukha
Svanasana)

4. Standing Forward
Bend (Uttanasana)

5. Chair Pose
(Utkatasana)

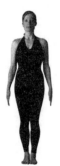

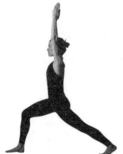

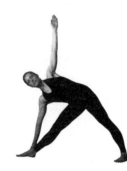
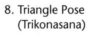

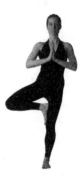

6. Mountain Pose
(Tadasana)

7. High Lunge (Alana)

8. Triangle Pose
(Trikonasana)

9. Tree Pose (Vrksasana)

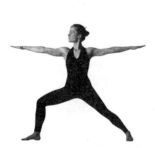

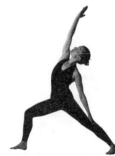

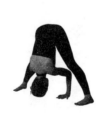

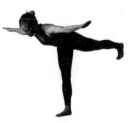

10. Warrior Pose II
(Virabhadrasana II)

11. Crescent Pose
(Virabhadrasana II
Variation)

12. Fan Pose (Prasarita
Padottanasana)

13. Warrior Pose III
(Virabhadrasana III)

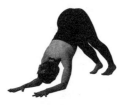

14. Forearm Stand Prep (Pincha Mayurasana Prep)

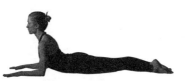

15. Sphinx Pose (Ardha Bhujangasana)

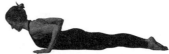

16. Cobra Pose (Bhujangasana)

17. Bridge Pose (Setu Bandha Sarvangasana)

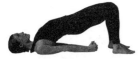

18. Shoulderstand Prep (Salamba Sarvangasana Prep)

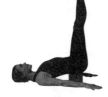

19. Maltese Twist (Jathara Parivartanasana)

1–5 Minutes

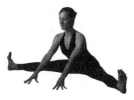

20. Seated Forward Bend (Paschimottanasana)

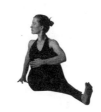

21. Seated Wide Angle Pose (Upavista Konasana)

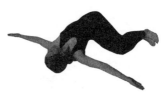

22. Seated Spinal Twist (Ardha Matsyendrasana)

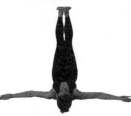

23. Energy Reversal Pose (Viparita Karani)

5–20 Minutes

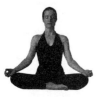

24. Seated Meditation Pose (Sukhasana)

5–10 Minutes

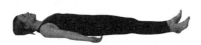

25. Corpse Pose (Savasana)

TEN-MINUTE CHAKRA FOCUS PRACTICES

Each of the following mini-practices can be used any time to balance the energy in a specific chakra.

Grounding: Muladhara

Mantra: LAM
Yantra: Golden square

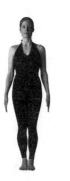

1. Mountain Pose
(Tadasana)

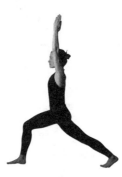

2. High Lunge
(Alana)

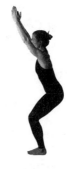

3. Chair Pose
(Utkatasana)

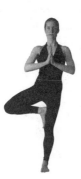

4. Tree Pose
(Vrksasana)

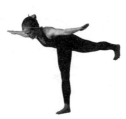

5. Warrior Pose III
(Virabhadrasana III)

Hip Opening: Svadhishthana

Mantra: VAM
Yantra: Silver crescent moon

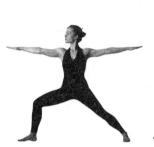
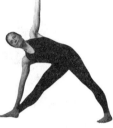

1. Warrior Pose II
   (Virabhadrasana II)

2. Triangle Pose
   (Trikonasana)

3. Fan Pose (Prasarita
   Padottanasana)

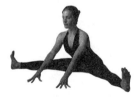
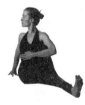

4. Seated Wide Angle Pose
   (Upavista Konasana)

5. Seated Spinal Twist
   (Ardha Matsyen-
   drasana)

Core Strength and Twisting: Manipura

Mantra: RAM
Yantra: Red triangle pointing down

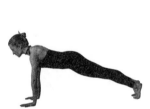

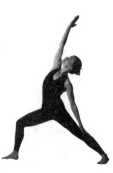

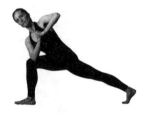

1. Incline Plank Pose (Ardha Chaturanga Dandasana)

2. Crescent Pose (Virabhadrasana II Variation)

3. Revolved Right Angle Pose (Parivrtta Parsvakonasana)

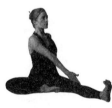

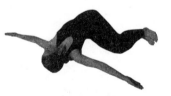

4. Revolved Head-to-Knee Pose (Parivrtta Janu Sirsasana)

5. Maltese Twist (Jathara Parivartanasana)

Back Bending: Anahata

Mantra: YAM
Yantra: Powder blue Star of David

Inhale ⟵———————⟶ Exhale × 5

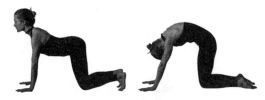

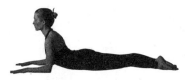

1–2. Upward-Facing Cat/Downward-Facing Cat
Pose (Marjariasana)

3. Sphinx Pose (Ardha
Bhujangasana)

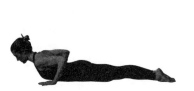

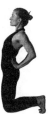

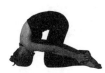

4. Cobra Pose
(Bhujangasana)

5. Camel Pose
(Ustrasana)

6. Hare Pose
(Hasangasana)

Shoulder Opening: Vishuddha

Mantra: VAM
Yantra: Egg shape

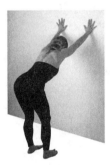

1. Arm Extension
   at the Wall

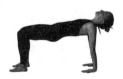

2. Downward-Facing Dog
   Pose (Adho Mukha
   Svanasana)

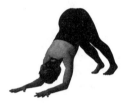

3. Forearm Stand Prep
   (Pincha Mayurasana
   Prep)

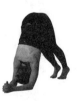

4. Headstand Prep
   (Sirsasana Prep)

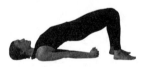

5. Four-Legged Table
   Pose (Chatushpada
   Pitham)

6. Bridge Pose
   (Setu Bandha
   Sarvangasana)

Ajna

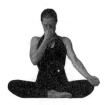

Alternate Nostril
Breathing (Nadi
Shodana Pranayama)

Full Relaxation: Sahasrara

Corpse Pose (Savasana)

RESOURCES

IF YOU WOULD LIKE to take a class with Alan or learn more about teacher training and the ISHTA system, please contact:

ISHTA Yoga
56 East 11th Street
New York, NY 10003
(212) 518-4800
www.ishtayoga.com

If you would like to learn more about chakra retreats and workshops with Katrina, please visit *www.katrinarepka.com.*